2. Turkey and Avocado Wrap

Ingredient:

- 4 whole wheat tortillas or wraps
- 8 oz sliced turkey breast
- 1 avocado, sliced
- 1 cup baby spinach or arugula
- 1/4 cup shredded carrots
- 2 tbsp hummus
- 1 tbsp olive oil
- Salt and pepper to taste

Instructions:

1. Lay the tortillas or wraps out on a clean surface.

2. Spread 1/2 tbsp of hummus evenly over each tortilla.

3. Layer the turkey slices, avocado slices, spinach/arugula, and shredded carrots onto the center of each tortilla.

4. Drizzle 1/4 tbsp of olive oil over the fillings on each wrap.

5. Season with salt and pepper to taste.

6. Fold the bottom of the tortilla up over the fillings, then fold in the sides and continue rolling tightly into a wrap.

7. Slice the wraps in half diagonally, if desired.

8. Serve immediately or wrap in parchment paper or foil to enjoy later.

The combination of savory turkey, creamy avocado, and crunchy veggies makes this a delicious and satisfying wrap. Enjoy!

3. Greek Yogurt with Berries and Honey

Ingredient:

• 1 cup plain Greek yogurt
• 1 cup mixed berries (such as blueberries, raspberries, blackberries)
• 2 tbsp honey
• 1 tsp lemon zest (optional)

Instructions:

1. Scoop the Greek yogurt into a serving bowl or parfait glass.

2. Top the yogurt with the mixed berries.

3. Drizzle the honey over the top of the berries.

4. If desired, sprinkle the lemon zest over the top.

5. Serve immediately or refrigerate until ready to enjoy.

That's it! This simple and healthy snack or breakfast is packed with protein from the Greek yogurt, antioxidants from the berries, and natural sweetness from the honey.

The lemon zest adds a bright, citrusy note that complements the other flavors. Feel free to use any combination of fresh or frozen berries that you prefer.

This Greek yogurt parfait is a delicious and nutritious way to start your day or satisfy a sweet craving. Enjoy!

Welcome to ***"Healthy Cookbook for Teen Boys: Boost Your Energy with 115+ Balanced and Flavorful Dishes"!*** This cookbook is your go-to resource for delicious and nutritious meals designed specifically to support the active lifestyle of teenage boys. Whether you're an athlete, a scholar, or simply navigating the challenges of adolescence, this book is here to help you fuel your body with meals that are not only good for you but also taste great.

Why This Cookbook?

As a teenage boy, your body is going through rapid growth and development. It's crucial to provide it with the right nutrients to support your energy levels, physical activities, and overall well-being. This cookbook emphasizes balanced nutrition with recipes that are rich in vitamins, minerals, lean proteins, and healthy fats—everything you need to thrive during this important stage of life.

What You'll Find Inside

Inside this cookbook, you'll discover over 115 recipes carefully selected to appeal to teenage boys' tastes and nutritional needs. From hearty breakfasts that kick-start your day to satisfying lunches, energizing snacks, and wholesome dinners, each recipe is designed to be both flavorful and nourishing.

Key Features:

- ***Nutrient-Packed Recipes:*** Enjoy a variety of dishes that are packed with nutrients essential for growth and development.

- ***Easy-to-Follow Instructions:*** Each recipe comes with clear, step-by-step instructions to make cooking simple and enjoyable.

- ***Balanced Nutrition:*** Emphasizing whole foods and healthy ingredients, these recipes help you maintain a balanced diet.

- ***Quick and Convenient:*** Many recipes are designed to be quick and easy, perfect for busy schedules.

- ***Tips for Success:*** Learn helpful tips on meal planning, cooking techniques, and ingredient substitutions to make cooking even easier.

Sample Recipes:
1. Protein-Packed Breakfast Burrito
2. Grilled Chicken Salad with Avocado Dressing

3. Turkey and Quinoa Stuffed Bell Peppers
4. Mango and Kale Smoothie
5. Baked Salmon with Sweet Potato Wedges

Start Cooking!

Whether you're a novice in the kitchen or already enjoy cooking, "Healthy Cookbook for Teen Boys: Boost Your Energy with 115+ Balanced and Flavorful Dishes" is your guide to creating meals that support your active lifestyle. Get ready to explore new flavors, discover the joy of cooking, and fuel your body with delicious and nutritious food. Let's cook up a healthier future together!

1. Grilled Chicken Salad

Ingredient:

• 4 boneless, skinless chicken breasts
• 1 tbsp olive oil
• 1 tsp garlic powder
• 1 tsp dried oregano
• Salt and pepper to taste
• 8 cups mixed greens (such as romaine, spinach, arugula)
• 1 cup cherry tomatoes, halved
• 1/2 cucumber, sliced
• 1/4 red onion, thinly sliced
• 1/4 cup crumbled feta cheese
• 2 tbsp balsamic vinaigrette

Instructions:

1. Preheat grill or grill pan to medium•high heat.

2. Brush the chicken breasts with olive oil and season with garlic powder, oregano, salt, and pepper.

3. Grill the chicken for 5•7 minutes per side, or until cooked through. Allow to cool slightly, then slice or chop the chicken.

4. In a large salad bowl, combine the mixed greens, tomatoes, cucumber, red onion, and feta cheese.

5. Top the salad with the grilled chicken. Drizzle the balsamic vinaigrette over the top and toss gently to coat. Serve immediately.

4. Oatmeal with Fresh Fruits and Nuts

Ingredient:

• 1 cup old•fashioned rolled oats
• 2 cups unsweetened almond milk (or milk of your choice)
• 1 tbsp honey (or maple syrup)
• 1/4 tsp ground cinnamon
• 1/4 tsp vanilla extract
• 1 cup mixed fresh fruit (such as sliced banana, berries, diced apple)
• 2 tbsp chopped nuts (such as almonds, walnuts, pecans)

Instructions:

1. In a medium saucepan, combine the rolled oats and almond milk. Bring to a simmer over medium heat, stirring occasionally.

2. Once the oats have thickened to your desired consistency, about 5•7 minutes, remove from heat.

3. Stir in the honey (or maple syrup), cinnamon, and vanilla extract. Mix well.

4. Transfer the oatmeal to a serving bowl.

5. Top the oatmeal with the mixed fresh fruit and chopped nuts.

6. Serve immediately, or cover and refrigerate for later.

This oatmeal dish is a nutritious and satisfying breakfast. The fresh fruits provide natural sweetness, fiber, and vitamins, while the nuts add healthy fats, protein, and crunch.

You can customize the toppings to your liking, using your favorite seasonal fruits and nuts. This is a great way to start your day with a balanced and delicious meal.

Enjoy your Oatmeal with Fresh Fruits and Nuts!

5. Quinoa Salad with Chickpeas and Veggies

Ingredient:

• 1 cup uncooked quinoa, rinsed
• 2 cups vegetable or chicken broth
• 1 (15 oz) can chickpeas, drained and rinsed
• 1 cup diced cucumber
• 1 cup cherry tomatoes, halved
• 1/2 cup diced red onion
• 1/2 cup crumbled feta cheese
• 2 tbsp chopped fresh parsley
• 2 tbsp olive oil
• 2 tbsp lemon juice
• 1 tsp Dijon mustard
• Salt and pepper to taste

Instructions:

1. In a medium saucepan, combine the quinoa and broth. Bring to a boil, then reduce heat to low, cover and simmer for 15•20 minutes, until quinoa is cooked and liquid is absorbed. Fluff with a fork and let cool.

2. In a large bowl, combine the cooked quinoa, chickpeas, cucumber, tomatoes, red onion, feta cheese, and parsley.

3. In a small bowl, whisk together the olive oil, lemon juice, and Dijon mustard. Season with salt and pepper.

4. Pour the dressing over the quinoa salad and toss gently to coat.

5. Serve chilled or at room temperature. Enjoy!

This quinoa salad is packed with protein, fiber, and fresh veggies. The chickpeas and feta add extra flavor and texture. You can customize the ingredients to your liking, such as adding other chopped vegetables or herbs.

This makes a great light and healthy lunch or side dish. It's also perfect for meal prepping and can be stored in the refrigerator for up to 4 days.

6. Whole Wheat Pasta with Marinara Sauce

Ingredient:

• 8 oz whole wheat pasta (such as spaghetti, penne, or fusilli)
• 1 tbsp olive oil
• 1 onion, diced
• 3 garlic cloves, minced
• 1 (28 oz) can crushed tomatoes
• 2 tbsp tomato paste
• 1 tsp dried oregano
• 1 tsp dried basil
• 1/4 tsp red pepper flakes (optional)
• Salt and pepper to taste
• Grated Parmesan cheese for serving (optional)

Instructions:

1. Bring a large pot of salted water to a boil. Cook the whole wheat pasta according to package instructions until al dente. Drain and set aside.

2. In a large skillet, heat the olive oil over medium heat. Add the diced onion and sauté for 5•7 minutes until translucent.

3. Add the minced garlic and cook for 1 minute until fragrant.

4. Pour in the crushed tomatoes and tomato paste. Stir in the dried oregano, basil, and red pepper flakes (if using). Season with salt and pepper to taste.

5. Simmer the marinara sauce for 10•15 minutes, stirring occasionally, until thickened slightly.

6. Add the cooked whole wheat pasta to the sauce and toss to coat evenly.

7. Serve the pasta warm, topped with grated Parmesan cheese if desired.

This whole wheat pasta dish is a healthier take on a classic Italian meal. The nutty, hearty whole wheat pasta pairs perfectly with the flavorful homemade marinara sauce. Feel free to add any extra vegetables or protein to make it a more complete meal.

Enjoy your Whole Wheat Pasta with Marinara Sauce!

7. Grilled Salmon with Steamed Broccoli

Ingredient:

- 4 (6 oz) salmon fillets
- 2 tbsp olive oil
- 1 tsp lemon zest
- 1 tbsp lemon juice
- 1 tsp dried dill
- Salt and pepper to taste
- 1 lb broccoli florets
- 2 tbsp water

Instructions:

1. Preheat grill or grill pan to medium•high heat.

2. In a small bowl, mix together the olive oil, lemon zest, lemon juice, and dried dill. Season the salmon fillets with salt and pepper, then brush the top of each fillet with the lemon•dill mixture.

3. Place the salmon fillets on the preheated grill or grill pan. Cook for 4•6 minutes per side, or until the salmon flakes easily with a fork and is cooked through.

4. While the salmon is grilling, place the broccoli florets in a steamer basket. Steam the broccoli for 5•7 minutes, until tender•crisp.

5. Remove the broccoli from the steamer and transfer to a serving bowl. Toss with 2 tbsp of water to keep it moist.

6. Serve the grilled salmon fillets immediately, alongside the steamed broccoli. Enjoy!

This simple yet delicious meal is packed with healthy omega•3 fatty acids from the salmon and fiber, vitamins, and minerals from the broccoli. The lemon•dill seasoning adds bright, fresh flavors to the salmon.

You can adjust the cooking time for the salmon based on your desired level of doneness. Pair this with a side salad or whole grain for a complete and balanced meal.

Enjoy your Grilled Salmon with Steamed Broccoli!

8. Veggie Stir•Fry with Tofu

Ingredient:

• 1 block (14 oz) extra•firm tofu, cubed
• 2 tbsp sesame oil, divided
• 2 cups mixed vegetables (such as broccoli florets, sliced bell peppers, snow peas, carrots)
• 1 cup sliced mushrooms
• 3 cloves garlic, minced
• 1 tbsp grated fresh ginger
• 2 tbsp low•sodium soy sauce
• 1 tbsp rice vinegar
• 1 tsp honey
• 1/4 tsp red pepper flakes (optional)
• Salt and pepper to taste
• Cooked brown rice, for serving

Instructions:

1. In a large skillet or wok, heat 1 tbsp of the sesame oil over medium•high heat. Add the cubed tofu and cook, stirring occasionally, until lightly browned on all sides, about 5•7 minutes. Transfer the tofu to a plate and set aside.

2. In the same skillet, heat the remaining 1 tbsp of sesame oil. Add the mixed vegetables and mushrooms. Stir•fry for 3•4 minutes until the vegetables are crisp•tender.

3. Add the minced garlic and grated ginger to the skillet. Cook for 1 minute, stirring constantly, until fragrant.

4. In a small bowl, whisk together the soy sauce, rice vinegar, and honey. Pour the sauce into the skillet and stir to coat the vegetables.

5. Add the cooked tofu back to the skillet and gently toss everything together. Cook for 2•3 minutes more, until the sauce has thickened slightly.

6. Remove from heat and season with salt, pepper, and red pepper flakes (if using).

7. Serve the veggie stir•fry immediately over cooked brown rice.

This colorful and flavorful veggie stir•fry is a delicious meatless meal. The tofu provides plant•based protein, while the variety of fresh vegetables add fiber, vitamins, and minerals. Adjust the vegetables based on your preferences.

9. Chicken and Vegetable Skewers

Ingredient:

• 1 lb boneless, skinless chicken breasts, cut into 1•inch cubes
• 1 red bell pepper, cut into 1•inch pieces
• 1 yellow bell pepper, cut into 1•inch pieces
• 1 zucchini, cut into 1/2•inch thick rounds
• 1 red onion, cut into 1•inch pieces
• 2 tbsp olive oil
• 2 tbsp lemon juice
• 1 tsp dried oregano
• 1 tsp garlic powder
• Salt and pepper to taste
• Wooden or metal skewers

Instructions:

1. In a large bowl, combine the cubed chicken, bell pepper pieces, zucchini rounds, and red onion pieces.

2. In a small bowl, whisk together the olive oil, lemon juice, oregano, and garlic powder. Season with salt and pepper.

3. Pour the marinade over the chicken and vegetables and toss to coat everything evenly. Cover and refrigerate for 30 minutes to 1 hour.

4. Preheat grill or grill pan to medium•high heat.

5. Thread the marinated chicken and vegetables onto the skewers, alternating the ingredients.

6. Grill the skewers for 12•15 minutes, turning occasionally, until the chicken is cooked through and the vegetables are tender.

7. Serve the grilled chicken and vegetable skewers immediately.

These colorful and flavorful skewers make a great main dish or appetizer. The marinade adds a zesty lemon•herb flavor that complements the grilled chicken and veggies.

You can use any combination of your favorite vegetables, such as mushrooms, cherry tomatoes, or pineapple chunks. Adjust the cooking time as needed based on the thickness of your chicken and vegetable pieces.

10. Brown Rice and Black Bean Bowl

Ingredient:

• 1 cup uncooked brown rice
• 1 (15 oz) can black beans, drained and rinsed
• 1 cup diced tomatoes
• 1/2 cup diced red onion
• 1 avocado, diced
• 2 tbsp chopped fresh cilantro
• 1 tbsp lime juice
• 1 tsp ground cumin
• 1/4 tsp chili powder
• Salt and pepper to taste

Instructions:

1. Cook the brown rice according to package instructions. Once cooked, fluff with a fork and set aside.

2. In a medium bowl, combine the drained and rinsed black beans, diced tomatoes, red onion, avocado, and chopped cilantro.

3. In a small bowl, whisk together the lime juice, cumin, chili powder, and a pinch of salt and pepper.

4. Pour the lime•spice dressing over the black bean and vegetable mixture. Toss gently to coat.

5. To assemble the bowls, divide the cooked brown rice evenly among 4 serving bowls. Top each portion of rice with the black bean and vegetable mixture.

6. Serve immediately, garnished with extra cilantro if desired.

This brown rice and black bean bowl is a nutritious and flavorful vegetarian meal. The combination of whole grains, protein•rich beans, fresh veggies, and zesty seasonings makes it a satisfying and balanced dish.

You can customize the toppings to your liking, such as adding shredded cheese, sour cream, or hot sauce. This recipe is also easily scalable if you want to meal prep it for the week.

Enjoy your delicious and wholesome Brown Rice and Black Bean Bowl!

11. Spinach and Mushroom Omelet

Ingredient:

• 3 eggs
• 1 tbsp milk or water
• 1 tsp olive oil
• 1/2 cup sliced mushrooms
• 1 cup fresh spinach leaves
• 2 tbsp shredded cheddar cheese
• Salt and pepper to taste

Instructions:

1. In a small bowl, whisk together the eggs and milk/water. Season with a pinch of salt and pepper.

2. Heat the olive oil in a small non•stick skillet over medium heat.

3. Add the sliced mushrooms to the skillet and sauté for 2•3 minutes until softened.

4. Add the fresh spinach leaves to the skillet and cook for 1 minute, stirring, until the spinach is wilted.

5. Pour the egg mixture into the skillet, tilting the pan to allow the uncooked egg to flow to the edges.

6. As the eggs start to set, use a spatula to gently push the cooked egg towards the center, tilting the pan to allow the uncooked egg to flow to the edges.

7. Once the eggs are mostly set but still a bit runny on top, sprinkle the shredded cheddar cheese over half of the omelet.

8. Fold the uncheesed half of the omelet over the cheesed half.

9. Slide the folded omelet onto a plate and serve immediately.

This spinach and mushroom omelet is a delicious and nutritious way to start your day. The fluffy eggs, sautéed veggies, and melty cheese make it a satisfying breakfast.

You can customize the fillings to your liking, such as adding diced tomatoes, bell peppers, or your favorite herbs. Serve with a side of whole grain toast or fresh fruit for a complete meal.

12. Beef and Vegetable Stir•Fry

Ingredient:
- 1 lb flank steak, thinly sliced against the grain
- 2 tbsp soy sauce, divided
- 1 tbsp cornstarch
- 2 tbsp vegetable oil, divided
- 3 cloves garlic, minced
- 1 tbsp grated fresh ginger
- 1 red bell pepper, sliced
- 1 cup broccoli florets
- 1 cup sliced mushrooms
- 1/2 cup sliced snow peas
- 2 tbsp oyster sauce
- 1 tbsp rice vinegar
- 1 tsp sesame oil
- Salt and pepper to taste
- Cooked brown rice, for serving

Instructions:
1. In a medium bowl, toss the sliced flank steak with 1 tbsp of soy sauce and the cornstarch until evenly coated.

2. Heat 1 tbsp of vegetable oil in a large skillet or wok over high heat. Add the marinated beef and stir•fry for 2•3 minutes until browned. Transfer the beef to a plate.

3. Add the remaining 1 tbsp of vegetable oil to the skillet. Stir in the minced garlic and grated ginger and cook for 1 minute until fragrant.

4. Add the sliced bell pepper, broccoli florets, mushrooms, and snow peas to the skillet. Stir•fry for 3•4 minutes until the vegetables are crisp•tender.

5. Return the cooked beef to the skillet. Add the remaining 1 tbsp of soy sauce, the oyster sauce, rice vinegar, and sesame oil. Toss everything together and cook for 2•3 minutes more.

6. Season the stir•fry with salt and pepper to taste. Serve the beef and vegetable stir•fry immediately over cooked brown rice.

This beef and vegetable stir•fry is a quick, healthy, and flavorful meal. The combination of tender beef, fresh veggies, and a savory sauce makes it a satisfying dish. Feel free to adjust the vegetables based on your preferences.

13. Tuna Salad with Whole Grain Crackers

Ingredient:

- 2 (5 oz) cans tuna, drained and flaked
- 2 tbsp plain Greek yogurt
- 1 tbsp mayonnaise
- 1 tbsp diced celery
- 1 tbsp diced red onion
- 1 tsp Dijon mustard
- 1 tsp lemon juice
- Salt and pepper to taste
- 8•10 whole grain crackers

Instructions:

1. In a medium bowl, combine the drained and flaked tuna, Greek yogurt, mayonnaise, celery, red onion, Dijon mustard, and lemon juice.

2. Mix everything together until well combined.

3. Season the tuna salad with salt and pepper to taste.

4. Serve the tuna salad with the whole grain crackers on the side.

This tuna salad is a nutritious and satisfying snack or light meal. The Greek yogurt and a small amount of mayonnaise help keep it creamy without adding too much fat. The celery and onion provide a nice crunch and flavor.

The whole grain crackers are a great accompaniment, providing a crunchy vehicle for the flavorful tuna salad. You can use your favorite whole grain crackers, such as whole wheat, multigrain, or even seeded crackers.

This tuna salad can also be served on top of mixed greens, stuffed into a tomato, or scooped onto cucumber slices for a low•carb option.

Enjoy your Tuna Salad with Whole Grain Crackers!

14. Lentil Soup

Ingredient:

- 1 tbsp olive oil
- 1 onion, diced
- 3 carrots, peeled and diced
- 3 celery stalks, diced
- 3 garlic cloves, minced
- 1 tsp ground cumin
- 1 tsp dried oregano
- 1/4 tsp red pepper flakes (optional)
- 1 cup dried brown or green lentils, rinsed
- 6 cups low•sodium vegetable or chicken broth
- 1 (14.5 oz) can diced tomatoes
- 2 bay leaves
- Salt and pepper to taste
- Chopped parsley for garnish (optional)

Instructions:

1. In a large pot or Dutch oven, heat the olive oil over medium heat. Add the diced onion, carrots, and celery. Sauté for 5•7 minutes until the vegetables are softened.

2. Stir in the minced garlic, cumin, oregano, and red pepper flakes (if using). Cook for 1 minute until fragrant.

3. Add the rinsed lentils, broth, diced tomatoes, and bay leaves. Bring the soup to a boil.

4. Reduce heat to low, cover, and simmer for 25•30 minutes, stirring occasionally, until the lentils are tender.

5. Remove the bay leaves. Season the soup with salt and pepper to taste.

6. Ladle the lentil soup into bowls and garnish with chopped parsley, if desired.

7. Serve hot, with crusty bread or a side salad.

This lentil soup is packed with fiber, protein, and nutrients from the lentils, vegetables, and herbs. It's a hearty, comforting, and satisfying meatless meal.

You can customize the soup by adding other vegetables like spinach, kale, or potatoes. For a creamier texture, you can blend a portion of the soup before serving.

15. Sweet Potato and Black Bean Tacos

Ingredient:

• 2 medium sweet potatoes, peeled and diced
• 1 tbsp olive oil
• 1 tsp chili powder
• 1/2 tsp ground cumin
• Salt and pepper to taste
• 1 (15 oz) can black beans, drained and rinsed
• 1 cup diced red onion
• 2 cloves garlic, minced
• 8•10 small corn or flour tortillas
• 1 avocado, sliced
• 1/4 cup crumbled feta or queso fresco
• Chopped cilantro for garnish

Instructions:

1. Preheat oven to 400°F. Toss the diced sweet potatoes with the olive oil, chili powder, cumin, salt, and pepper. Spread in a single layer on a baking sheet.

2. Roast the sweet potatoes for 20•25 minutes, stirring halfway, until tender and lightly browned.

3. In a skillet over medium heat, sauté the drained and rinsed black beans, diced red onion, and minced garlic for 3•4 minutes until fragrant.

4. To assemble the tacos, place a spoonful of the roasted sweet potatoes into each tortilla. Top with the black bean mixture, sliced avocado, crumbled feta or queso fresco, and chopped cilantro.

5. Serve the sweet potato and black bean tacos immediately.

These vegetarian tacos are full of flavor and nutrition. The sweet potatoes provide a natural sweetness that pairs perfectly with the savory black beans and tangy feta or queso fresco.

You can customize the toppings to your liking, such as adding diced tomatoes, shredded cabbage, or a drizzle of lime crema.

Enjoy your delicious Sweet Potato and Black Bean Tacos!

16. Cottage Cheese with Pineapple

Ingredient:
- 1 cup low•fat or non•fat cottage cheese
- 1/2 cup diced fresh pineapple
- 1 tsp honey (optional)

Instructions:

1. Scoop the cottage cheese into a small bowl or serving dish.

2. Top the cottage cheese with the diced pineapple.

3. If desired, drizzle the honey over the top of the pineapple.

4. Serve immediately.

That's it! This is a quick and easy snack or light breakfast that's packed with protein, vitamins, and natural sweetness.

The cottage cheese provides a creamy, high•protein base, while the fresh pineapple adds a bright, tropical flavor. The honey is optional, but can be added if you want a little extra sweetness.

You can adjust the amounts of each ingredient to suit your taste preferences. Some other variations include:

- Using crushed pineapple instead of diced
- Sprinkling a bit of cinnamon over the top
- Adding a sprinkle of toasted coconut or chopped nuts
- Using a different fruit like mango or berries instead of pineapple

This Cottage Cheese with Pineapple makes for a nutritious and satisfying snack or light meal. It's simple to prepare and perfect for a quick, healthy option.

Enjoy!

17. Grilled Shrimp with Asparagus

Ingredient:

• 1 lb large shrimp, peeled and deveined
• 1 lb asparagus, trimmed
• 2 tbsp olive oil, divided
• 1 tbsp lemon juice
• 2 tsp minced garlic
• 1 tsp dried oregano
• 1/2 tsp crushed red pepper flakes (optional)
• Salt and pepper to taste

Instructions:

1. In a large bowl, combine the shrimp, 1 tbsp of olive oil, lemon juice, minced garlic, oregano, and red pepper flakes (if using). Toss to coat the shrimp evenly. Season with salt and pepper.

2. In a separate bowl, toss the asparagus with the remaining 1 tbsp of olive oil and season with salt and pepper.

3. Preheat grill or grill pan to medium•high heat.

4. Thread the marinated shrimp onto metal or wooden skewers.

5. Grill the shrimp skewers and the asparagus for 3•5 minutes per side, or until the shrimp are opaque and the asparagus is tender•crisp.

6. Remove the shrimp and asparagus from the grill and transfer to a serving platter.

7. Serve the grilled shrimp and asparagus immediately, garnished with lemon wedges if desired.

This grilled shrimp and asparagus dish is a quick, healthy, and flavorful meal. The shrimp are marinated in a zesty garlic•herb mixture, while the asparagus gets a simple seasoning of olive oil, salt, and pepper.

You can adjust the amount of red pepper flakes to control the level of spice. Serve this dish with a side of rice, quinoa, or a fresh salad for a complete and balanced meal.

Enjoy your Grilled Shrimp with Asparagus!

18. Turkey Chili

Ingredient:

- 1 lb ground turkey
- 1 onion, diced
- 3 cloves garlic, minced
- 2 tbsp chili powder
- 1 tsp ground cumin
- 1 tsp dried oregano
- 1/2 tsp smoked paprika
- 1/4 tsp cayenne pepper (optional)
- 1 (15 oz) can diced tomatoes
- 1 (15 oz) can kidney beans, drained and rinsed
- 1 (15 oz) can black beans, drained and rinsed
- 1 cup low·sodium chicken or vegetable broth
- Salt and pepper to taste
- Toppings (e.g. shredded cheese, diced avocado, chopped cilantro)

Instructions:

1. In a large pot or Dutch oven, cook the ground turkey over medium·high heat, breaking it up with a wooden spoon, until browned and cooked through, about 5·7 minutes. Drain any excess fat.

2. Add the diced onion to the pot and cook for 3·4 minutes until softened. Stir in the minced garlic and cook for 1 minute until fragrant.

3. Add the chili powder, cumin, oregano, smoked paprika, and cayenne (if using). Stir to coat the turkey and vegetables.

4. Pour in the diced tomatoes, kidney beans, black beans, and chicken/vegetable broth. Stir to combine.

5. Bring the chili to a simmer, then reduce heat to low. Let the chili simmer for 20·25 minutes, stirring occasionally, until thickened.

6. Season the chili with salt and pepper to taste.

7. Serve the turkey chili hot, topped with your desired toppings such as shredded cheese, diced avocado, and chopped cilantro.

This turkey chili is a healthier, leaner alternative to traditional beef chili. The combination of ground turkey, beans, and spices creates a flavorful and satisfying meal.

You can adjust the spice level by adding more or less cayenne pepper. Serve the chili with cornbread, tortilla chips, or a side salad for a complete and nourishing dinner.

Enjoy your Turkey Chili!

19. Hummus and Veggie Wrap

Ingredient:

• 4 whole wheat tortillas or wraps
• 1 cup hummus
• 1 cup shredded carrots
• 1 cup sliced cucumber
• 1 cup baby spinach or arugula
• 1/2 cup diced red bell pepper
• 2 tbsp crumbled feta cheese (optional)

Instructions:

1. Spread about 1/4 cup of hummus evenly over each whole wheat tortilla or wrap.

2. Arrange the shredded carrots, sliced cucumber, baby spinach/arugula, and diced red bell pepper in the center of each tortilla.

3. If using, sprinkle the crumbled feta cheese over the vegetables.

4. Fold the bottom of the tortilla up over the fillings, then fold in the sides and continue rolling tightly into a wrap.

5. Slice the wraps in half diagonally, if desired.

6. Serve the hummus and veggie wraps immediately, or wrap them in parchment paper or foil to enjoy later.

These hummus and veggie wraps make for a delicious and nutritious meal or snack. The creamy hummus provides a protein•rich base, while the fresh vegetables add crunch, flavor, and fiber.

You can customize the fillings to your liking, using your favorite veggies such as avocado, tomatoes, or mushrooms. The feta cheese adds a tangy flavor, but you can omit it for a dairy•free option.

These wraps are perfect for meal prepping or packing for lunch. Enjoy your Hummus and Veggie Wrap!

20. Chicken and Quinoa Stuffed Peppers

Ingredient:

• 4 bell peppers, halved lengthwise and seeds removed
• 1 cup cooked quinoa
• 1 cup cooked and shredded chicken breast
• 1 (15 oz) can black beans, drained and rinsed
• 1 cup diced tomatoes
• 1/2 cup shredded cheddar cheese
• 2 tbsp chopped fresh cilantro
• 1 tsp ground cumin
• 1/2 tsp chili powder
• Salt and pepper to taste

Instructions:

1. Preheat oven to 375°F. Place the bell pepper halves in a baking dish and set aside.

2. In a large bowl, combine the cooked quinoa, shredded chicken, black beans, diced tomatoes, 1/4 cup of the shredded cheddar cheese, cilantro, cumin, and chili powder. Season with salt and pepper.

3. Spoon the chicken and quinoa mixture evenly into the bell pepper halves, packing it in gently.

4. Top the stuffed peppers with the remaining 1/4 cup of shredded cheddar cheese.

5. Cover the baking dish with foil and bake for 25•30 minutes, until the peppers are tender.

6. Remove the foil and bake for an additional 5 minutes to melt and brown the cheese on top.

7. Serve the Chicken and Quinoa Stuffed Peppers warm.

These stuffed peppers are a nutritious and flavorful meal. The combination of protein•rich chicken, fiber•filled quinoa, and nutrient•dense vegetables makes it a well•balanced dish.

You can customize the filling by using different types of beans, adding sautéed onions or garlic, or using a different type of cheese. Serve the stuffed peppers with a side salad or roasted vegetables for a complete meal.

21. Almond Butter and Banana Sandwich on Whole Grain Bread

Ingredient:

• 2 slices whole grain bread
• 2 tbsp creamy almond butter
• 1 ripe banana, sliced

Instructions:

1. Spread the almond butter evenly on one slice of the whole grain bread.

2. Arrange the sliced banana over the almond butter in a single layer.

3. Place the second slice of whole grain bread on top to create a sandwich.

4. Cut the sandwich in half diagonally, if desired.

That's it! This simple sandwich makes for a delicious and nutritious snack or light meal.

The combination of creamy almond butter and sweet banana is a classic flavor pairing. The whole grain bread provides complex carbohydrates, fiber, and additional nutrients.

Some variations you could try:

• Use crunchy almond butter instead of creamy
• Add a drizzle of honey or maple syrup
• Sprinkle a pinch of cinnamon over the banana slices
• Use a different nut or seed butter, such as peanut butter or sunflower seed butter
• Toast the bread before assembling the sandwich

This Almond Butter and Banana Sandwich is a quick, easy, and satisfying way to enjoy a wholesome, balanced snack. It's perfect for a grab•and•go breakfast or a midday pick•me•up.

Enjoy!

22. Baked Cod with Lemon and Dill

Ingredient:

• 1 lb cod fillets
• 2 tbsp olive oil
• 2 tbsp freshly squeezed lemon juice
• 2 tsp dried dill
• 1 tsp grated lemon zest
• Salt and pepper to taste
• Lemon wedges for serving

Instructions:

1. Preheat your oven to 400°F (200°C).

2. Place the cod fillets in a baking dish or on a parchment•lined baking sheet.

3. In a small bowl, whisk together the olive oil, lemon juice, dried dill, and lemon zest.

4. Drizzle the lemon•dill mixture over the cod fillets, making sure to evenly coat the fish.

5. Season the cod with salt and pepper to taste.

6. Bake the cod in the preheated oven for 12•15 minutes, or until the fish is opaque and flakes easily with a fork.

7. Serve the baked cod immediately, garnished with lemon wedges.

This simple baked cod recipe is a delicious and healthy way to enjoy white fish. The bright flavors of lemon and dill complement the mild taste of the cod perfectly.

You can adjust the cooking time based on the thickness of your cod fillets. Thicker pieces may require a few extra minutes in the oven.

Serve the baked cod with roasted vegetables, a fresh salad, or steamed rice for a complete and balanced meal. Enjoy your Baked Cod with Lemon and Dill!

23. Veggie Burger with a Side Salad

Ingredient:

Veggie Burgers:
• 4 veggie burger patties (store•bought or homemade)
• 4 whole wheat buns or lettuce wraps
• Toppings of your choice (e.g. tomato, onion, pickles, avocado, etc.)

Side Salad:
• 4 cups mixed greens (e.g. spinach, arugula, romaine)
• 1 cup cherry tomatoes, halved
• 1/2 cucumber, sliced
• 1/4 red onion, thinly sliced
• 2 tbsp olive oil
• 1 tbsp balsamic vinegar
• Salt and pepper to taste

Instructions:

Veggie Burgers:
1. Cook the veggie burger patties according to package instructions or your homemade recipe.
2. Toast the whole wheat buns (or prepare the lettuce wraps).
3. Place the cooked veggie burger patty on the bottom bun (or lettuce wrap).
4. Top with your desired toppings.
5. Place the top bun (or close the lettuce wrap) and serve immediately.

Side Salad:
1. In a large salad bowl, combine the mixed greens, cherry tomatoes, cucumber, and red onion.
2. Drizzle the olive oil and balsamic vinegar over the salad.
3. Season with salt and pepper to taste.
4. Toss the salad gently to coat with the dressing.

To serve, place the veggie burger on a plate and accompany it with the side salad.

This meal provides a balance of plant•based protein from the veggie burger and a fresh, nutrient•dense side salad. The combination of the hearty veggie burger and the crisp, flavorful salad makes for a satisfying and wholesome meal.

Feel free to customize the veggie burger toppings and salad ingredients to your liking. Enjoy your Veggie Burger with a Side Salad!

24. Smoothie with Spinach, Banana, and Almond Milk

Ingredient:

• 1 cup unsweetened almond milk
• 1 cup fresh spinach leaves
• 1 ripe banana, frozen
• 1 tbsp almond butter
• 1 tsp honey (optional)
• 1/2 tsp vanilla extract
• Ice cubes (optional)

Instructions:

1. In a high•powered blender, combine the unsweetened almond milk, fresh spinach leaves, frozen banana, almond butter, honey (if using), and vanilla extract.

2. Blend on high speed until the mixture is smooth and creamy, about 1•2 minutes.

3. If you'd like a thicker, colder smoothie, add a few ice cubes and blend again until the desired consistency is reached.

4. Pour the smoothie into a glass and enjoy immediately.

This spinach, banana, and almond milk smoothie is a nutritious and delicious way to start your day. The spinach provides a boost of vitamins and minerals, while the banana and almond butter add natural sweetness and creaminess.

The almond milk serves as the base, making this smoothie dairy•free and plant•based. The honey is optional, but can be added if you prefer a sweeter taste.

You can customize this smoothie by using different types of nut butters, adding other fruits like berries or mango, or even incorporating a scoop of protein powder.

Enjoy your refreshing and healthy Spinach, Banana, and Almond Milk Smoothie!

25. Egg and Avocado Breakfast Burrito

Ingredient:

• 4 eggs, scrambled
• 1 avocado, diced
• 1/4 cup diced tomatoes
• 2 tbsp diced red onion
• 1 tbsp chopped cilantro
• 1 tsp hot sauce (optional)
• Salt and pepper to taste
• 4 whole wheat tortillas or wraps

Instructions:

1. In a medium skillet, scramble the eggs over medium heat until cooked through. Season with salt and pepper.

2. In a small bowl, combine the diced avocado, tomatoes, red onion, and chopped cilantro. Season with a pinch of salt and pepper.

3. Lay the whole wheat tortillas or wraps out on a clean surface.

4. Divide the scrambled eggs evenly among the tortillas, placing them in the center.

5. Top the eggs with the avocado•vegetable mixture.

6. If using, drizzle a small amount of hot sauce over the fillings.

7. Fold the bottom of the tortilla up over the fillings, then fold in the sides and continue rolling tightly into a burrito.

8. Serve the egg and avocado breakfast burritos immediately, or wrap them in parchment paper or foil to enjoy later.

These breakfast burritos are a nutritious and satisfying way to start your day. The combination of protein•rich eggs, creamy avocado, and fresh vegetables makes for a well•balanced meal.

You can customize the fillings by adding other ingredients like shredded cheese, sautéed spinach, or diced bell peppers. The hot sauce adds a nice kick of flavor, but it's optional.

Enjoy your Egg and Avocado Breakfast Burrito!

26. Chicken and Veggie Stir•Fry

Ingredient:

• 1 lb boneless, skinless chicken breasts, cut into 1•inch pieces
• 2 tbsp soy sauce, divided
• 1 tbsp cornstarch
• 2 tbsp sesame oil, divided
• 3 cloves garlic, minced
• 1 tbsp grated fresh ginger
• 1 red bell pepper, sliced
• 1 cup broccoli florets
• 1 cup sliced mushrooms
• 1 cup snow peas
• 2 tbsp rice vinegar
• 1 tsp honey
• Salt and pepper to taste
• Cooked brown rice, for serving

Instructions:

1. In a medium bowl, toss the chicken pieces with 1 tbsp of soy sauce and the cornstarch until evenly coated.

2. Heat 1 tbsp of sesame oil in a large skillet or wok over high heat. Add the chicken and stir•fry for 3•4 minutes until lightly browned. Transfer the chicken to a plate.

3. Add the remaining 1 tbsp of sesame oil to the skillet. Stir in the minced garlic and grated ginger, and cook for 1 minute until fragrant.

4. Add the sliced bell pepper, broccoli florets, mushrooms, and snow peas to the skillet. Stir•fry for 4•5 minutes until the vegetables are crisp•tender.

5. Return the cooked chicken to the skillet. Add the remaining 1 tbsp of soy sauce, rice vinegar, and honey. Toss everything together and cook for 2•3 minutes more.

6. Season the stir•fry with salt and pepper to taste. Serve the chicken and veggie stir•fry immediately over cooked brown rice.

This colorful and flavorful stir•fry is a quick and healthy meal. The combination of tender chicken, fresh vegetables, and a savory sauce makes it a satisfying dish.

Feel free to substitute or add other vegetables based on your preferences. Adjust the cooking time as needed to ensure the chicken is cooked through and the vegetables are at your desired doneness

27. Whole Grain Pancakes with Fresh Berries

Ingredient:

• 1 cup whole wheat flour
• 1 tsp baking powder
• 1/2 tsp baking soda
• 1/4 tsp salt
• 1 cup unsweetened almond milk (or milk of your choice)
• 1 egg
• 1 tbsp honey
• 1 tsp vanilla extract
• 1 cup fresh berries (such as blueberries, raspberries, or sliced strawberries)
• Maple syrup for serving (optional)

Instructions:

1. In a medium bowl, whisk together the whole wheat flour, baking powder, baking soda, and salt.

2. In a separate bowl, whisk together the almond milk, egg, honey, and vanilla extract.

3. Pour the wet ingredients into the dry ingredients and stir just until combined (do not overmix).

4. Heat a lightly oiled non•stick skillet or griddle over medium heat.

5. Scoop about 1/4 cup of the pancake batter onto the hot skillet. Cook for 2•3 minutes, or until bubbles start to form on the surface.

6. Flip the pancake and cook for an additional 1•2 minutes, until golden brown.

7. Repeat with the remaining batter, making about 12 pancakes total.

8. Serve the whole grain pancakes warm, topped with the fresh berries and a drizzle of maple syrup, if desired.

These whole grain pancakes are a nutritious and delicious breakfast option. The combination of nutty whole wheat flour, sweet berries, and a touch of honey makes them satisfying and flavorful.

You can use any type of fresh or frozen berries you prefer. Adjust the amount of honey based on the sweetness of your berries.

28. Beef and Bean Burrito Bowl

Ingredient:

- 1 lb ground beef
- 1 onion, diced
- 3 cloves garlic, minced
- 1 tbsp chili powder
- 1 tsp ground cumin
- 1/2 tsp dried oregano
- Salt and pepper to taste
- 1 (15 oz) can black beans, drained and rinsed
- 1 cup cooked brown rice
- 1 cup diced tomatoes
- 1 avocado, diced
- 1/4 cup shredded cheddar cheese
- 2 tbsp chopped fresh cilantro
- Lime wedges for serving

Instructions:

1. In a large skillet over medium•high heat, cook the ground beef, breaking it up with a wooden spoon, until browned and cooked through, about 5•7 minutes. Drain any excess fat.

2. Add the diced onion to the skillet and cook for 3•4 minutes until softened. Stir in the minced garlic and cook for 1 minute until fragrant.

3. Season the beef mixture with the chili powder, cumin, oregano, salt, and pepper. Stir to combine.

4. Add the drained and rinsed black beans to the skillet and heat through, about 2•3 minutes.

5. To assemble the burrito bowls, divide the cooked brown rice evenly among 4 serving bowls. Top each bowl with the beef and bean mixture, diced tomatoes, diced avocado, shredded cheddar cheese, and chopped cilantro.

6. Serve the burrito bowls immediately, with lime wedges on the side for squeezing over the top.

This Beef and Bean Burrito Bowl is a delicious and satisfying meal. The seasoned ground beef and black beans provide protein, while the brown rice, tomatoes, avocado, and cilantro add fiber, vitamins, and fresh flavors.

You can customize the toppings to your liking, such as adding sour cream, salsa, or jalapeños. This recipe is also easily scalable if you want to meal prep it for the week.

29. Tomato and Cucumber Salad with Feta

Ingredient:

• 2 cups cherry or grape tomatoes, halved
• 1 English cucumber, sliced
• 1/2 red onion, thinly sliced
• 1/2 cup crumbled feta cheese
• 2 tbsp olive oil
• 1 tbsp red wine vinegar
• 1 tbsp fresh lemon juice
• 1 tsp dried oregano
• Salt and black pepper to taste
• Fresh chopped basil or parsley for garnish (optional)

Instructions:

1. In a large bowl, combine the halved tomatoes, sliced cucumber, and sliced red onion.

2. In a small bowl, whisk together the olive oil, red wine vinegar, lemon juice, and dried oregano. Season with salt and pepper to taste.

3. Pour the dressing over the tomato, cucumber and onion mixture. Toss gently to coat.

4. Sprinkle the crumbled feta cheese over the top of the salad.

5. Garnish with fresh chopped basil or parsley, if desired.

6. Refrigerate for at least 30 minutes to allow the flavors to meld.

7. Serve chilled or at room temperature.

This simple salad is full of fresh, vibrant flavors from the juicy tomatoes, crisp cucumbers, tangy feta and zesty dressing. It makes a great side dish or light main course. Enjoy!

30. Grilled Chicken and Avocado Salad

Ingredient:

• 2 boneless, skinless chicken breasts
• 1 tbsp olive oil
• Salt and pepper to taste
• 8 cups mixed greens (such as spinach, arugula, romaine)
• 1 avocado, diced
• 1 cup cherry tomatoes, halved
• 1/4 cup thinly sliced red onion
• 2 tbsp crumbled feta cheese
• 2 tbsp balsamic vinaigrette

Instructions:

1. Preheat grill or grill pan to medium•high heat.

2. Brush the chicken breasts with olive oil and season generously with salt and pepper.

3. Grill the chicken for 5•7 minutes per side, until cooked through. Allow to rest for 5 minutes, then slice or chop the chicken.

4. In a large salad bowl, combine the mixed greens, diced avocado, cherry tomatoes, and sliced red onion.

5. Top the salad with the grilled chicken slices.

6. Sprinkle the crumbled feta cheese over the top.

7. Drizzle the balsamic vinaigrette over the salad and toss gently to coat.

8. Serve immediately.

The combination of juicy grilled chicken, creamy avocado, fresh veggies, and tangy feta makes this salad incredibly flavorful and satisfying. Feel free to adjust the ingredient amounts to your taste. Enjoy!

31. Lentil and Vegetable Stew

Ingredient:

- 1 cup dry brown or green lentils, rinsed
- 4 cups vegetable broth
- 1 tbsp olive oil
- 1 onion, diced
- 3 cloves garlic, minced
- 2 carrots, peeled and diced
- 2 celery stalks, diced
- 1 bell pepper, diced
- 1 (14.5 oz) can diced tomatoes
- 2 tsp dried thyme
- 1 tsp dried oregano
- Salt and black pepper to taste
- Chopped fresh parsley for garnish (optional)

Instructions:

1. In a large pot, combine the lentils and vegetable broth. Bring to a boil over high heat.

2. Reduce heat to medium•low, cover and simmer for 15•20 minutes, until lentils are tender.

3. In a separate large pot or Dutch oven, heat the olive oil over medium heat.

4. Add the onion and garlic and cook for 2•3 minutes until fragrant.

5. Add the carrots, celery, and bell pepper. Cook for 5•7 minutes, stirring occasionally, until vegetables are tender.

6. Stir in the cooked lentils, diced tomatoes, thyme, oregano, salt and pepper.

7. Bring the stew to a simmer and cook for 10•15 minutes, allowing the flavors to meld.

8. Taste and adjust seasonings as needed.

9. Serve hot, garnished with chopped fresh parsley if desired.

This hearty, nutritious stew is packed with fiber, protein and veggies. It makes a satisfying meatless main dish. Enjoy!

32. Turkey and Spinach Meatballs

Ingredient:
• 1 lb ground turkey
• 1 cup fresh spinach, finely chopped
• 1/2 cup breadcrumbs
• 1/4 cup grated Parmesan cheese
• 2 cloves garlic, minced
• 1 egg
• 1 tsp dried oregano
• 1/2 tsp salt
• 1/4 tsp black pepper

For Serving:
• Marinara sauce
• Whole wheat pasta or zucchini noodles

Instructions:

1. Preheat oven to 400°F. Line a baking sheet with parchment paper.

2. In a large bowl, combine the ground turkey, chopped spinach, breadcrumbs, Parmesan, garlic, egg, oregano, salt and pepper. Mix well until fully incorporated.

3. Scoop the mixture and roll into 1•inch meatballs, placing them on the prepared baking sheet.

4. Bake for 18•20 minutes, until the meatballs are cooked through and lightly browned.

5. Meanwhile, warm the marinara sauce in a saucepan over medium heat.

6. Serve the turkey and spinach meatballs over whole wheat pasta or zucchini noodles, topped with the warm marinara sauce.

The spinach adds moisture and nutrients to these lean turkey meatballs. They make a delicious, healthy main dish or appetizer. Enjoy!

33. Greek Salad with Grilled Chicken

Ingredient:

Salad:
• 6 cups chopped romaine lettuce
• 1 cup cherry tomatoes, halved
• 1 cucumber, diced
• 1/2 red onion, thinly sliced
• 1/2 cup pitted kalamata olives, halved
• 1/2 cup crumbled feta cheese

Dressing:
• 2 tbsp olive oil
• 1 tbsp red wine vinegar
• 1 tbsp lemon juice
• 1 tsp Dijon mustard
• 1 tsp dried oregano
• Salt and pepper to taste

Grilled Chicken:
• 1 lb boneless, skinless chicken breasts
• 1 tbsp olive oil
• 1 tsp dried oregano
• 1/2 tsp garlic powder
• Salt and pepper to taste

Instructions:

1. Preheat grill or grill pan to medium•high heat.

2. In a small bowl, combine the olive oil, dried oregano, garlic powder, salt, and pepper. Rub the mixture all over the chicken breasts.

3. Grill the chicken for 5•7 minutes per side, or until cooked through. Allow to rest for 5 minutes, then slice or chop the chicken.

4. In a large salad bowl, combine the chopped romaine, cherry tomatoes, diced cucumber, sliced red onion, and kalamata olives.

5. In a small bowl, whisk together the olive oil, red wine vinegar, lemon juice, Dijon mustard, dried oregano, salt, and pepper to make the dressing.

6. Add the grilled chicken and crumbled feta cheese to the salad. Drizzle the dressing over the top and toss gently to coat. Serve the Greek Salad with Grilled Chicken immediately.

This colorful and flavorful salad is a complete meal, featuring protein•rich grilled chicken, fresh vegetables, and a tangy Greek•inspired dressing. The combination of flavors and textures makes it a delicious and satisfying option.

Feel free to adjust the amounts of the salad ingredients to your liking. You can also add other toppings like pepperoncini, chickpeas, or fresh herbs.

34. Broccoli and Cheddar Stuffed Potatoes

Ingredient:

- 4 medium russet potatoes
- 1 cup broccoli florets, steamed and chopped
- 1/2 cup shredded cheddar cheese
- 2 tbsp milk
- 2 tbsp butter
- 1/4 tsp salt
- 1/8 tsp black pepper
- 2 tbsp chopped green onions (optional)

Instructions:

1. Preheat oven to 400°F. Wash the potatoes and prick them several times with a fork.

2. Bake the potatoes directly on the oven rack for 50·60 minutes, until tender when pierced with a fork.

3. Remove the potatoes from the oven and let cool for 5 minutes. Cut each potato in half lengthwise.

4. Scoop the potato flesh into a medium bowl, leaving a thin layer of potato attached to the skin.

5. Add the steamed and chopped broccoli, shredded cheddar cheese, milk, butter, salt and pepper to the potato flesh. Mash and stir until well combined.

6. Spoon the broccoli and cheddar potato mixture back into the potato skins.

7. Place the stuffed potato halves back on the baking sheet.

8. Bake for an additional 10·15 minutes, until the cheese is melted and lightly browned on top.

9. Garnish with chopped green onions, if desired.

Serve these hearty, cheesy stuffed potatoes as a main dish or side. Enjoy!

35. Shrimp and Veggie Stir•Fry

Ingredient:

• 1 lb large shrimp, peeled and deveined
• 2 tbsp sesame oil
• 2 cloves garlic, minced
• 1 inch piece fresh ginger, grated
• 1 red bell pepper, sliced
• 1 cup broccoli florets
• 1 cup snow peas or snap peas
• 1/2 cup sliced mushrooms
• 2 tbsp low•sodium soy sauce
• 1 tbsp rice vinegar
• 1 tsp honey
• 1/4 tsp red pepper flakes (optional)
• Salt and pepper to taste
• Cooked brown rice, for serving

Instructions:

1. In a large skillet or wok, heat the sesame oil over medium•high heat.

2. Add the shrimp, garlic, and ginger. Stir•fry for 2•3 minutes until the shrimp start to turn pink.

3. Add the sliced bell pepper, broccoli, snow peas, and mushrooms. Stir•fry for 4•5 minutes until the vegetables are tender•crisp.

4. In a small bowl, whisk together the soy sauce, rice vinegar, and honey.

5. Pour the sauce into the skillet and toss everything together. Cook for 1•2 minutes until the sauce thickens slightly.

6. Remove from heat and season with salt, pepper, and red pepper flakes if desired.

7. Serve the shrimp and veggie stir•fry immediately over cooked brown rice.

This quick and easy stir•fry is packed with protein, fiber, and fresh flavors. Adjust the vegetables based on your preferences. Enjoy!

36. Apple Slices with Peanut Butter

Ingredient:

• 1 medium apple, cored and sliced
• 2•3 tbsp creamy peanut butter

Instructions:

1. Wash and slice the apple into thin wedges or slices.

2. Arrange the apple slices on a plate or platter.

3. Scoop the peanut butter into a small bowl or ramekin.

4. Serve the apple slices alongside the peanut butter for dipping.

That's it! This makes a quick, nutritious, and satisfying snack or light dessert.

The crisp, juicy apple pairs perfectly with the creamy, protein•rich peanut butter. You can use any variety of apple you prefer • Gala, Fuji, Honeycrisp, etc.

For added flavor, you can sprinkle a pinch of cinnamon over the apple slices before serving. You can also try using almond butter or another nut butter instead of peanut butter.

This simple snack is a great way to satisfy a sweet craving while getting some beneficial nutrients from the fruit and healthy fats from the nut butter. Enjoy!

37. Grilled Vegetable Sandwich

Ingredient:

• 1 zucchini, sliced lengthwise into 1/4·inch thick strips
• 1 red bell pepper, sliced into 1/2·inch thick strips
• 1 eggplant, sliced into 1/2·inch thick rounds
• 1 red onion, sliced into 1/2·inch thick rings
• 2 tbsp olive oil
• Salt and pepper to taste
• 8 slices whole grain bread
• 4 oz crumbled feta cheese
• 2 tbsp pesto (store·bought or homemade)

Instructions:

1. Preheat grill or grill pan to medium·high heat.

2. In a large bowl, toss the zucchini, bell pepper, eggplant, and red onion slices with the olive oil. Season with salt and pepper.

3. Grill the vegetables for 3·5 minutes per side, or until they are tender and have grill marks.

4. Remove the grilled vegetables from the grill and let them cool slightly.

5. Spread 1 tbsp of pesto on 4 slices of the whole grain bread.

6. Top the pesto·coated bread slices with the grilled vegetables, dividing them evenly.

7. Sprinkle the crumbled feta cheese over the vegetables.

8. Place the remaining 4 slices of bread on top to create the sandwiches.

9. Grill the sandwiches for 2·3 minutes per side, or until the bread is toasted and the cheese is melted. Serve the grilled vegetable sandwiches immediately.

This grilled vegetable sandwich is a delicious and nutritious meatless option. The combination of tender, flavorful grilled veggies, creamy feta, and fragrant pesto makes for a satisfying and flavorful meal.

You can customize the vegetables used based on your preferences. The pesto can also be substituted with other spreads, such as hummus or roasted red pepper spread.

38. Chicken and Brown Rice Soup

Ingredient:

- 1 tbsp olive oil
- 1 onion, diced
- 3 carrots, peeled and sliced
- 3 celery stalks, sliced
- 3 cloves garlic, minced
- 6 cups low•sodium chicken broth
- 1 cup cooked brown rice
- 2 cups shredded cooked chicken
- 1 tsp dried thyme
- 1 bay leaf
- Salt and pepper to taste
- Chopped fresh parsley for garnish (optional)

Instructions:

1. In a large pot or Dutch oven, heat the olive oil over medium heat.

2. Add the diced onion, sliced carrots, and sliced celery. Cook for 5•7 minutes, stirring occasionally, until the vegetables start to soften.

3. Stir in the minced garlic and cook for 1 minute until fragrant.

4. Pour in the chicken broth and add the cooked brown rice, shredded chicken, dried thyme, and bay leaf.

5. Bring the soup to a simmer and let it cook for 15•20 minutes, allowing the flavors to meld.

6. Remove the bay leaf. Season the soup with salt and pepper to taste.

7. Ladle the chicken and brown rice soup into bowls. Garnish with chopped fresh parsley if desired.

This hearty, nourishing soup is perfect for a chilly day. The combination of tender chicken, chewy brown rice, and fresh vegetables makes it a satisfying meal. Enjoy!

39. Spaghetti Squash with Marinara Sauce

Ingredient:

• 1 medium spaghetti squash
• 1 tbsp olive oil
• 1 jar (24 oz) marinara sauce
• 1/4 cup grated Parmesan cheese (optional)
• Fresh basil leaves, chopped (optional)

Instructions:

1. Preheat oven to 400°F. Cut the spaghetti squash in half lengthwise and scoop out the seeds.

2. Brush the inside of the squash halves with the olive oil. Place the squash halves cut•side down on a baking sheet.

3. Bake for 40•50 minutes, until the squash is tender and can be easily shredded with a fork.

4. Remove the squash from the oven and let cool slightly. Use a fork to shred the flesh of the squash into spaghetti•like strands.

5. In a saucepan, heat the marinara sauce over medium heat until warmed through.

6. Divide the spaghetti squash strands between plates or bowls. Top each serving with the warm marinara sauce.

7. Sprinkle with Parmesan cheese and chopped fresh basil, if desired.

Enjoy this healthy, low•carb alternative to traditional pasta! The spaghetti squash provides a similar texture and the marinara sauce adds classic Italian flavor.

40. Grilled Salmon Tacos

Ingredient:

- 1 lb salmon fillets
- 2 tbsp olive oil
- 1 tsp chili powder
- 1 tsp cumin
- 1/2 tsp garlic powder
- Salt and pepper to taste
- 8•10 small corn or flour tortillas
- 1 cup shredded cabbage or slaw mix
- 1 avocado, diced
- 1/4 cup crumbled feta cheese
- Lime wedges for serving

For the Chipotle Crema:
- 1/2 cup plain Greek yogurt
- 2 tbsp mayonnaise
- 1 chipotle pepper in adobo sauce, finely chopped
- 1 tbsp lime juice
- 1/4 tsp salt

Instructions:

1. Preheat grill or grill pan to medium•high heat.

2. In a small bowl, mix together the olive oil, chili powder, cumin, garlic powder, salt and pepper. Brush this seasoning mixture over the salmon fillets.

3. Grill the salmon for 4•6 minutes per side, until cooked through and flaky. Remove from heat and flake the salmon into chunks.

4. In a small bowl, make the chipotle crema by combining the Greek yogurt, mayonnaise, chopped chipotle pepper, lime juice and salt. Stir well.

5. Warm the tortillas according to package instructions.

6. To assemble the tacos, place some of the grilled salmon chunks into each tortilla. Top with shredded cabbage, diced avocado, and a drizzle of the chipotle crema.

7. Sprinkle crumbled feta cheese over the top. Serve the salmon tacos immediately with lime wedges on the side.

The smoky, spiced salmon pairs perfectly with the cool, creamy chipotle crema and fresh toppings. Enjoy these tasty grilled salmon tacos!

41. Cottage Cheese and Mixed Fruit

Ingredient:

• 1 cup low•fat or non•fat cottage cheese
• 1 cup mixed fresh fruit (such as berries, diced apple, diced mango, etc.)
• 1•2 tsp honey or maple syrup (optional)

Instructions:

1. Scoop the cottage cheese into a bowl.

2. Top the cottage cheese with the mixed fresh fruit.

3. If desired, drizzle a small amount of honey or maple syrup over the top.

4. Gently stir to combine.

That's it! This makes a quick, healthy, and delicious snack or light meal. The cottage cheese provides protein, while the fruit adds natural sweetness and fiber. Feel free to use your favorite combination of fresh fruits. Enjoy!

42. Chicken Caesar Salad with a Light Dressing

Ingredient:

For the Salad:
• 4 cups chopped romaine lettuce
• 2 cups cooked, shredded chicken breast
• 1/2 cup croutons
• 2 tbsp grated Parmesan cheese

For the Light Caesar Dressing:
• 1/4 cup plain Greek yogurt
• 2 tbsp lemon juice
• 1 tbsp Dijon mustard
• 1 garlic clove, minced
• 1 tsp Worcestershire sauce
• 2 tbsp olive oil
• Salt and pepper to taste

Instructions:

1. In a medium bowl, whisk together all the ingredients for the light Caesar dressing • the Greek yogurt, lemon juice, Dijon mustard, garlic, Worcestershire sauce, olive oil, salt and pepper. Set aside.

2. In a large salad bowl, combine the chopped romaine lettuce, shredded cooked chicken, croutons, and grated Parmesan cheese.

3. Drizzle the light Caesar dressing over the salad and toss gently to coat.

4. Serve the Chicken Caesar Salad immediately.

The light Caesar dressing is made with Greek yogurt instead of mayonnaise or heavy cream, cutting down on calories and fat. The combination of crisp romaine, lean chicken, crunchy croutons, and tangy dressing makes this a satisfying and nutritious salad.

You can adjust the amounts of each ingredient to suit your taste preferences. Enjoy this healthier take on a classic Chicken Caesar Salad!

43. Baked Ziti with Whole Wheat Pasta

Ingredient:

• 8 oz whole wheat ziti or penne pasta
• 1 lb lean ground turkey or ground beef
• 1 onion, diced
• 3 cloves garlic, minced
• 1 (28 oz) can crushed tomatoes
• 1 (6 oz) can tomato paste
• 1 tsp dried oregano
• 1 tsp dried basil
• 1/2 tsp red pepper flakes (optional)
• Salt and pepper to taste
• 1 cup part•skim ricotta cheese
• 1 cup shredded part•skim mozzarella cheese
• 1/4 cup grated Parmesan cheese

Instructions:

1. Preheat oven to 375°F. Grease a 9x13 inch baking dish.

2. Bring a large pot of salted water to a boil. Cook the whole wheat pasta according to package instructions until al dente. Drain and set aside.

3. In a large skillet, cook the ground turkey or beef over medium•high heat, breaking it up as it cooks, until browned, about 5•7 minutes. Drain any excess fat.

4. Add the diced onion and minced garlic to the skillet. Cook for 2•3 minutes until fragrant.

5. Stir in the crushed tomatoes, tomato paste, oregano, basil, red pepper flakes (if using), and season with salt and pepper. Simmer for 5•10 minutes.

6. In a large bowl, combine the cooked pasta, meat sauce, ricotta cheese, 1/2 cup of the mozzarella cheese, and 2 tbsp of the Parmesan cheese. Mix well.

7. Transfer the pasta mixture to the prepared baking dish. Top with the remaining 1/2 cup mozzarella and 2 tbsp Parmesan cheese.

8. Bake for 20•25 minutes, until the cheese is melted and lightly browned on top.

9. Let stand for 5 minutes before serving.

44. Tuna and Avocado Salad

Ingredient:

- 2 (5 oz) cans tuna, drained
- 1 ripe avocado, diced
- 2 tbsp plain Greek yogurt
- 1 tbsp lemon juice
- 1 tbsp finely chopped red onion
- 2 tsp Dijon mustard
- 1 tsp dried dill (or 1 tbsp fresh dill)
- Salt and pepper to taste
- Lettuce leaves or whole grain bread/crackers, for serving

Instructions:

1. In a medium bowl, gently mix together the drained tuna, diced avocado, Greek yogurt, lemon juice, red onion, Dijon mustard, and dried dill.

2. Season the tuna and avocado salad with salt and pepper to taste.

3. Serve the tuna and avocado salad on a bed of lettuce leaves, or use it as a spread on whole grain bread or crackers.

This simple salad is packed with healthy fats from the avocado, protein from the tuna, and a creamy dressing made with Greek yogurt. The lemon juice, Dijon, and dill add a nice tangy and herbal flavor.

You can adjust the amounts of each ingredient to your taste preferences. For extra crunch, you can also add chopped celery, cucumber, or toasted nuts.

This tuna and avocado salad makes a great light lunch or snack. Enjoy!

45. Sweet Potato and Turkey Hash

Ingredient:

- 2 medium sweet potatoes, peeled and diced
- 1 lb ground turkey
- 1 onion, diced
- 2 cloves garlic, minced
- 1 red bell pepper, diced
- 1 tsp smoked paprika
- 1 tsp dried thyme
- 1/4 tsp cayenne pepper (optional)
- Salt and black pepper to taste
- 2 tbsp olive oil
- 2 eggs (optional)

Instructions:

1. In a large skillet or cast iron pan, heat the olive oil over medium•high heat.

2. Add the diced sweet potatoes and cook for 8•10 minutes, stirring occasionally, until they start to soften.

3. Add the ground turkey, diced onion, minced garlic, and diced bell pepper to the pan. Cook for 5•7 minutes, breaking up the turkey as it cooks, until the turkey is browned and the vegetables are tender.

4. Stir in the smoked paprika, dried thyme, cayenne (if using), and season with salt and pepper to taste.

5. Continue cooking the hash for 5•7 more minutes, allowing the flavors to meld and the sweet potatoes to become tender.

6. If desired, create 2 wells in the hash and crack the eggs into them. Cover the pan and cook the eggs to your desired doneness.

7. Serve the sweet potato and turkey hash immediately, with the fried eggs on top if using.

This hearty, flavorful hash makes a wonderful breakfast, brunch or even dinner. The sweet potatoes, turkey, and spices create a delicious combination. Enjoy!

46. Veggie and Cheese Quesadilla

Ingredient:

• 4 whole wheat tortillas
• 1 cup shredded cheddar or Monterey Jack cheese
• 1 cup diced bell peppers (any color)
• 1/2 cup sliced mushrooms
• 1/2 cup diced onion
• 1 cup baby spinach leaves
• 1 tbsp olive oil
• Salt and pepper to taste

Optional Toppings:
• Salsa
• Guacamole
• Sour cream
• Chopped cilantro

Instructions:

1. Heat a large skillet or griddle over medium heat. Brush the surface lightly with olive oil.

2. Place one tortilla in the skillet. On half of the tortilla, layer 1/4 cup of the shredded cheese, 1/4 cup of the diced bell peppers, 2 tbsp of the sliced mushrooms, 2 tbsp of the diced onion, and a handful of the baby spinach leaves.

3. Fold the other half of the tortilla over the filled half to create a half•moon shape.

4. Cook the quesadilla for 2•3 minutes per side, until the tortilla is lightly golden brown and the cheese is melted.

5. Repeat steps 2•4 with the remaining 3 tortillas and fillings.

6. Cut each quesadilla in half and serve immediately, with desired toppings on the side.

These veggie•packed quesadillas make a quick and easy meatless meal or snack. The combination of melty cheese, fresh veggies, and whole wheat tortillas is both satisfying and nutritious. Enjoy!

47. Chicken and Spinach Wrap

Ingredient:

• 2 cups cooked, shredded chicken breast
• 2 cups fresh spinach leaves
• 1/2 cup shredded mozzarella cheese
• 2 tbsp low•fat cream cheese, softened
• 1 tbsp Dijon mustard
• 1 tsp dried oregano
• Salt and pepper to taste
• 4 whole wheat tortillas or wraps

Instructions:

1. In a medium bowl, combine the shredded chicken, spinach, mozzarella cheese, cream cheese, Dijon mustard, and dried oregano. Season with salt and pepper to taste. Mix well until fully incorporated.

2. Lay the tortillas or wraps out on a clean surface. Divide the chicken and spinach mixture evenly among the 4 wraps, placing it in the center of each one.

3. Fold the bottom of the wrap up over the filling, then fold in the sides and continue rolling up tightly into a burrito shape.

4. Heat a large skillet or griddle over medium heat. Place the wrapped sandwiches seam•side down in the pan and cook for 2•3 minutes per side, until lightly golden brown.

5. Remove the wraps from the heat and slice in half diagonally, if desired.

6. Serve the chicken and spinach wraps immediately, while warm.

These wraps make a great portable lunch or light dinner. The combination of lean protein, fresh greens, and melty cheese is both satisfying and nutritious. Enjoy!

48. Quinoa and Black Bean Salad

Ingredient:

• 1 cup uncooked quinoa, rinsed
• 1 (15 oz) can black beans, drained and rinsed
• 1 cup diced cucumber
• 1 cup diced tomatoes
• 1/2 cup diced red onion
• 1/4 cup chopped fresh cilantro
• 2 tbsp olive oil
• 2 tbsp lime juice
• 1 tsp ground cumin
• 1/2 tsp chili powder
• Salt and pepper to taste

Instructions:

1. Cook the quinoa according to package instructions. Allow to cool completely.

2. In a large bowl, combine the cooked and cooled quinoa, black beans, diced cucumber, tomatoes, red onion, and chopped cilantro.

3. In a small bowl, whisk together the olive oil, lime juice, cumin, and chili powder. Season with salt and pepper.

4. Pour the dressing over the quinoa and bean salad and toss gently to coat.

5. Refrigerate the salad for at least 30 minutes to allow the flavors to meld.

6. Serve chilled or at room temperature.

This quinoa and black bean salad is packed with protein, fiber, and fresh veggies. It makes a great side dish or light main course. The zesty lime dressing complements the earthy quinoa and beans perfectly. Enjoy!

49. Grilled Steak with a Side Salad

Ingredient:

For the Steak:
• 1 lb flank steak or skirt steak
• 2 tbsp olive oil
• 2 tsp garlic powder
• 1 tsp dried oregano
• Salt and pepper to taste

For the Salad:
• 5 cups mixed greens (such as spinach, arugula, romaine)
• 1 cup cherry tomatoes, halved
• 1/2 cucumber, sliced
• 1/4 red onion, thinly sliced
• 2 tbsp crumbled feta cheese
• 2 tbsp balsamic vinaigrette

Instructions:

For the Steak:
1. Pat the steak dry with paper towels and season both sides generously with the garlic powder, oregano, salt, and pepper.
2. Heat a grill or grill pan over medium•high heat. Brush the grill grates with olive oil.
3. Grill the steak for 4•6 minutes per side, depending on thickness, until it reaches your desired doneness.
4. Transfer the grilled steak to a cutting board and let it rest for 5 minutes before slicing against the grain.

For the Salad:
1. In a large salad bowl, combine the mixed greens, cherry tomatoes, cucumber slices, and red onion.
2. Drizzle the balsamic vinaigrette over the salad and toss gently to coat.
3. Sprinkle the crumbled feta cheese over the top.

To Serve:
1. Arrange the sliced grilled steak on a plate or platter.
2. Serve the side salad alongside the steak.

This simple yet satisfying meal features juicy grilled steak paired with a fresh, flavorful side salad. Enjoy!

50. Hummus with Carrot and Celery Sticks

Ingredient:

• 1 (15 oz) can chickpeas (garbanzo beans), drained and rinsed
• 2 tbsp tahini (sesame seed paste)
• 2 tbsp fresh lemon juice
• 1 garlic clove, minced
• 2 tbsp olive oil
• 1/4 tsp ground cumin
• 1/4 tsp paprika
• Salt and pepper to taste
• 4•5 carrots, peeled and cut into sticks
• 4•5 celery stalks, cut into sticks

Instructions:

1. In a food processor or high•powered blender, combine the drained and rinsed chickpeas, tahini, lemon juice, garlic, olive oil, cumin, and paprika. Blend until smooth and creamy.

2. Taste the hummus and season with salt and pepper as needed. You can also add a bit more lemon juice, olive oil, or spices to adjust the flavor to your liking.

3. Transfer the hummus to a serving bowl or plate.

4. Arrange the carrot and celery sticks around the edges of the hummus.

5. Serve immediately, or refrigerate until ready to serve.

This classic hummus dip is packed with protein, fiber, and healthy fats from the chickpeas and tahini. The fresh veggies provide a satisfying crunch and extra nutrients. Enjoy this simple, nutritious snack!

51. Egg Salad on Whole Grain Toast

Ingredient:

• 6 hard boiled eggs, peeled and chopped
• 2 tbsp plain Greek yogurt
• 1 tbsp Dijon mustard
• 1 tbsp finely chopped celery
• 1 tbsp finely chopped red onion
• 1 tsp lemon juice
• 1/4 tsp salt
• 1/8 tsp black pepper
• 4 slices whole grain bread, toasted

Instructions:

1. In a medium bowl, combine the chopped hard boiled eggs, Greek yogurt, Dijon mustard, celery, red onion, lemon juice, salt, and pepper. Mix well until fully incorporated.

2. Toast the whole grain bread slices until lightly golden brown.

3. Divide the egg salad evenly among the 4 toast slices, spreading it over the surface.

4. Serve the egg salad toasts immediately.

This egg salad is made with a lighter dressing of Greek yogurt instead of mayonnaise, cutting down on calories and fat. The addition of crunchy celery, onion, and tangy Dijon adds great flavor.

You can serve the egg salad on toasted whole grain bread, or use it as a dip for veggie sticks, crackers, or lettuce wraps. It also makes a great sandwich filling.

This protein•packed egg salad is a nutritious and satisfying option for breakfast, lunch, or a snack. Enjoy!

52. Chicken and Vegetable Soup

Ingredient:

- 1 tbsp olive oil
- 1 onion, diced
- 3 carrots, peeled and sliced
- 3 celery stalks, sliced
- 3 cloves garlic, minced
- 6 cups low•sodium chicken broth
- 2 cups shredded cooked chicken
- 1 cup frozen peas
- 1 cup frozen corn
- 1 tsp dried thyme
- 1 bay leaf
- Salt and pepper to taste
- Chopped fresh parsley for garnish (optional)

Instructions:

1. In a large pot or Dutch oven, heat the olive oil over medium heat.

2. Add the diced onion, sliced carrots, and sliced celery. Cook for 5•7 minutes, stirring occasionally, until the vegetables start to soften.

3. Stir in the minced garlic and cook for 1 minute until fragrant.

4. Pour in the chicken broth and add the shredded cooked chicken, frozen peas, frozen corn, dried thyme, and bay leaf.

5. Bring the soup to a simmer and let it cook for 15•20 minutes, allowing the flavors to meld.

6. Remove the bay leaf. Season the soup with salt and pepper to taste.

7. Ladle the chicken and vegetable soup into bowls. Garnish with chopped fresh parsley if desired.

This hearty, nourishing soup is packed with lean protein, fresh vegetables, and comforting flavors. It makes a satisfying meal on its own or served with crusty bread. Enjoy!

53. Baked Tilapia with Green Beans

Ingredient:

• 4 tilapia fillets (about 1 lb total)
• 1 lb fresh green beans, trimmed
• 2 tbsp olive oil, divided
• 1 tsp garlic powder
• 1 tsp dried oregano
• 1/2 tsp paprika
• Salt and pepper to taste
• 1 lemon, cut into wedges (for serving)

Instructions:

1. Preheat oven to 400°F. Line a large baking sheet with parchment paper.

2. In a large bowl, toss the trimmed green beans with 1 tbsp of the olive oil. Season with salt and pepper.

3. Spread the green beans out in a single layer on one side of the prepared baking sheet.

4. In a small bowl, mix together the garlic powder, oregano, paprika, and a pinch of salt and pepper.

5. Rub the remaining 1 tbsp of olive oil over both sides of the tilapia fillets. Sprinkle the seasoning mixture evenly over the fish.

6. Place the seasoned tilapia fillets on the other side of the baking sheet, next to the green beans.

7. Bake for 15•18 minutes, until the fish flakes easily with a fork and the green beans are tender.

8. Serve the baked tilapia and green beans immediately, with lemon wedges on the side.

This simple one•pan meal is healthy, quick, and delicious. The tilapia is flaky and flavorful, while the roasted green beans provide a nutritious side. Enjoy!

54. Greek Yogurt with Granola and Honey

Ingredient:

- 1 cup plain Greek yogurt
- 1/2 cup granola
- 2 tbsp honey

Instructions:

1. Scoop the Greek yogurt into a bowl or parfait glass.

2. Sprinkle the granola evenly over the top of the yogurt.

3. Drizzle the honey over the granola.

That's it! This simple, 3•ingredient snack or breakfast is both nutritious and satisfying.

The creamy Greek yogurt provides protein and probiotics. The crunchy granola adds fiber, complex carbs, and healthy fats. And the sweet honey ties it all together.

You can use any type of granola you prefer • store•bought or homemade. For extra flavor, you can also add fresh fruit like berries, sliced bananas, or diced apples.

This Greek yogurt parfait is a great way to start your day or enjoy a healthy snack. The combination of tangy yogurt, sweet honey, and nutty granola is simply delicious. Enjoy!

55. Turkey and Veggie Stir•Fry

Ingredient:

• 1 lb ground turkey
• 2 tbsp sesame oil
• 2 cloves garlic, minced
• 1 inch fresh ginger, grated
• 1 red bell pepper, sliced
• 1 cup broccoli florets
• 1 cup snow peas
• 1 cup sliced mushrooms
• 2 tbsp low•sodium soy sauce
• 1 tbsp rice vinegar
• 1 tsp honey
• Salt and pepper to taste
• Cooked brown rice, for serving

Instructions:

1. In a large skillet or wok, heat the sesame oil over medium•high heat.

2. Add the ground turkey and cook, breaking it up with a spatula, until browned and cooked through, about 5•7 minutes.

3. Add the minced garlic and grated ginger to the skillet. Cook for 1 minute until fragrant.

4. Stir in the sliced red bell pepper, broccoli florets, snow peas, and mushrooms. Cook for 4•5 minutes, until the vegetables are tender•crisp.

5. In a small bowl, whisk together the soy sauce, rice vinegar, and honey.

6. Pour the sauce into the skillet and toss everything together. Cook for 1•2 minutes until the sauce thickens slightly.

7. Remove from heat and season with salt and pepper to taste.

8. Serve the turkey and veggie stir•fry immediately over cooked brown rice.

This quick and easy stir•fry is packed with lean protein, fresh produce, and bold Asian•inspired flavors. Adjust the vegetables based on your preferences. Enjoy!

56. Cottage Cheese with Tomatoes and Cucumbers

Ingredient:

- 1 cup low•fat or non•fat cottage cheese
- 1 cup cherry or grape tomatoes, halved
- 1 cup diced cucumber
- 1 tbsp chopped fresh basil (or 1 tsp dried basil)
- 1 tsp olive oil
- 1 tsp balsamic vinegar
- Salt and pepper to taste

Instructions:

1. In a medium bowl, combine the cottage cheese, halved tomatoes, and diced cucumber.

2. Drizzle the olive oil and balsamic vinegar over the top.

3. Sprinkle the chopped fresh basil (or dried basil) over the salad.

4. Season with salt and pepper to taste.

5. Gently toss the ingredients together until well combined.

6. Serve immediately or refrigerate until ready to enjoy.

This simple cottage cheese salad is a refreshing and nutritious snack or light meal. The cool, creamy cottage cheese pairs perfectly with the juicy tomatoes, crunchy cucumbers, and aromatic basil.

You can adjust the amounts of each ingredient to your taste preferences. For extra flavor, you can also add a sprinkle of feta cheese or a squeeze of lemon juice.

This cottage cheese salad is a great source of protein, fiber, and vitamins. Enjoy it as a healthy and satisfying option any time of day.

57. Baked Sweet Potato Fries

Ingredient:

• 2 medium sweet potatoes, peeled and cut into 1/2•inch thick fry shapes
• 2 tbsp olive oil
• 1 tsp paprika
• 1/2 tsp garlic powder
• 1/2 tsp salt
• 1/4 tsp black pepper

Instructions:

1. Preheat oven to 400°F. Line a large baking sheet with parchment paper.

2. In a large bowl, toss the sweet potato fry shapes with the olive oil, paprika, garlic powder, salt, and pepper until evenly coated.

3. Spread the seasoned sweet potato fries in a single layer on the prepared baking sheet, making sure they are not touching each other.

4. Bake for 20•25 minutes, flipping the fries halfway through, until they are tender and lightly browned.

5. Remove the baked sweet potato fries from the oven and serve immediately.

These baked sweet potato fries are a healthier alternative to traditional fried potatoes. The natural sweetness of the sweet potatoes pairs perfectly with the savory spices.

You can adjust the seasonings to your taste preferences. Try adding a pinch of cayenne pepper for a little heat, or sprinkle on some grated Parmesan cheese when they come out of the oven.

Serve these crispy, oven•baked sweet potato fries as a side dish or a nutritious snack. Enjoy!

58. Beef and Vegetable Kabobs

Ingredient:
• 1 lb beef sirloin or tenderloin, cut into 1•inch cubes
• 1 red bell pepper, cut into 1•inch pieces
• 1 yellow bell pepper, cut into 1•inch pieces
• 1 red onion, cut into 1•inch pieces
• 8 oz mushrooms, halved
• 2 zucchini, cut into 1•inch pieces
• 2 tbsp olive oil
• 2 tsp dried oregano
• 1 tsp garlic powder
• Salt and pepper to taste
• Wooden or metal skewers

For the Marinade:
• 1/4 cup low•sodium soy sauce
• 2 tbsp lemon juice
• 1 tbsp honey
• 2 cloves garlic, minced
• 1 tsp ground ginger

Instructions:

1. In a shallow dish, whisk together all the marinade ingredients. Add the beef cubes and toss to coat. Cover and refrigerate for 30 minutes to 1 hour.

2. Preheat grill or grill pan to medium•high heat.

3. Thread the marinated beef, bell peppers, onion, mushrooms, and zucchini onto the skewers, alternating the ingredients.

4. In a small bowl, mix together the olive oil, oregano, garlic powder, salt and pepper.

5. Brush the kabobs with the seasoned oil mixture.

6. Grill the kabobs for 10•12 minutes, turning occasionally, until the beef is cooked through and the vegetables are tender.

7. Serve the beef and vegetable kabobs immediately.

These colorful kabobs are packed with lean protein, fresh produce, and bold flavors from the marinade and seasoning. Enjoy them as a main dish or appetizer.

59. Lentil and Spinach Salad

Ingredient:

- 1 cup cooked lentils, cooled
- 4 cups fresh spinach leaves, chopped
- 1 cup cherry tomatoes, halved
- 1/2 cup diced cucumber
- 1/4 cup crumbled feta cheese
- 2 tbsp olive oil
- 1 tbsp balsamic vinegar
- 1 tsp Dijon mustard
- 1 clove garlic, minced
- Salt and pepper to taste

Instructions:

1. In a large salad bowl, combine the cooked and cooled lentils, chopped spinach, halved cherry tomatoes, and diced cucumber.

2. In a small bowl, whisk together the olive oil, balsamic vinegar, Dijon mustard, and minced garlic. Season with salt and pepper.

3. Pour the dressing over the lentil and spinach salad and toss gently to coat.

4. Sprinkle the crumbled feta cheese over the top of the salad.

5. Serve immediately or refrigerate until ready to enjoy.

This lentil and spinach salad is packed with protein, fiber, vitamins, and healthy fats. The lentils provide a hearty base, while the fresh spinach, tomatoes, and cucumber add crunch and freshness. The tangy balsamic dressing ties all the flavors together.

You can customize this salad by adding other veggies, nuts, or seeds. It makes a great main dish or side salad. Enjoy this nutritious and delicious lentil and spinach creation!

60. Chicken and Quinoa Bowl

Ingredient:

• 1 cup uncooked quinoa, rinsed
• 2 cups low•sodium chicken broth
• 1 lb boneless, skinless chicken breasts
• 1 tbsp olive oil
• 1 tsp garlic powder
• 1 tsp dried oregano
• Salt and pepper to taste
• 1 cup diced cucumber
• 1 cup cherry tomatoes, halved
• 1/4 cup crumbled feta cheese
• 2 tbsp chopped fresh parsley
• 1 tbsp lemon juice

Instructions:

1. In a medium saucepan, combine the rinsed quinoa and chicken broth. Bring to a boil, then reduce heat to low, cover and simmer for 15•20 minutes until quinoa is tender. Fluff with a fork and set aside.

2. Preheat oven to 400°F. Season the chicken breasts with the garlic powder, oregano, salt and pepper.

3. Heat the olive oil in a large oven•safe skillet over medium•high heat. Add the seasoned chicken and sear for 2•3 minutes per side until browned.

4. Transfer the skillet to the preheated oven and bake for 15•18 minutes, until the chicken is cooked through. Allow to rest for 5 minutes, then slice or shred the chicken.

5. In a large bowl, combine the cooked quinoa, sliced or shredded chicken, diced cucumber, halved cherry tomatoes, crumbled feta, and chopped parsley.

6. Drizzle the lemon juice over the top and gently toss to combine.

7. Serve the chicken and quinoa bowl immediately.

This nutritious and satisfying bowl is full of lean protein, whole grains, fresh veggies, and bold flavors. Enjoy!

61. Apple and Cheddar Sandwich

Ingredient:

• 2 slices whole grain or multigrain bread
• 2 tbsp creamy peanut butter (or almond butter)
• 1 small apple, thinly sliced
• 2 oz sharp cheddar cheese, sliced

Instructions:

1. Spread the peanut butter (or almond butter) evenly on one slice of bread.

2. Layer the thinly sliced apple over the peanut butter.

3. Top the apple slices with the cheddar cheese slices.

4. Place the remaining slice of bread on top to create a sandwich.

5. Heat a skillet or griddle over medium heat.

6. Place the sandwich in the skillet and cook for 2•3 minutes per side, until the bread is lightly toasted and the cheese is melted.

7. Remove the sandwich from the heat and slice in half diagonally, if desired.

8. Serve the apple and cheddar sandwich immediately.

The combination of crisp apple, creamy peanut butter, and melty cheddar cheese makes this a delightful and satisfying sandwich. The whole grain bread adds fiber and nutrients.

You can use any variety of apple that you prefer. Granny Smith or Honeycrisp work especially well. Feel free to adjust the amount of peanut butter or cheese to your taste.

This apple and cheddar sandwich makes a great lunch or snack. Enjoy!

62. Grilled Tuna Steak with Asparagus

Ingredient:

• 4 tuna steaks (about 6 oz each)
• 1 lb asparagus, trimmed
• 2 tbsp olive oil
• 2 tbsp lemon juice
• 1 tsp dried oregano
• Salt and pepper to taste

Instructions:

1. Preheat grill to medium•high heat.

2. In a shallow dish, combine the olive oil, lemon juice, oregano, salt and pepper. Add the tuna steaks and turn to coat both sides.

3. Grill the tuna steaks for 3•4 minutes per side, or until cooked to your desired doneness. Transfer to a plate and cover to keep warm.

4. In the same dish, toss the asparagus with the remaining marinade.

5. Grill the asparagus for 5•7 minutes, turning occasionally, until tender•crisp.

6. Serve the grilled tuna steaks immediately, topped with the grilled asparagus.

Enjoy your healthy and delicious grilled tuna and asparagus meal!

63. Vegetable and Bean Chili

Ingredient:

• 1 tbsp olive oil
• 1 onion, diced
• 3 cloves garlic, minced
• 1 red bell pepper, diced
• 1 zucchini, diced
• 1 can (15 oz) black beans, drained and rinsed
• 1 can (15 oz) kidney beans, drained and rinsed
• 1 can (28 oz) diced tomatoes
• 2 tbsp chili powder
• 1 tsp ground cumin
• 1 tsp dried oregano
• 1/2 tsp smoked paprika
• Salt and pepper to taste
• Chopped cilantro for garnish (optional)

Instructions:

1. In a large pot or Dutch oven, heat the olive oil over medium heat. Add the onion and sauté for 5 minutes until translucent.

2. Add the garlic, bell pepper, and zucchini. Cook for 3•4 minutes, stirring occasionally, until the vegetables start to soften.

3. Stir in the black beans, kidney beans, diced tomatoes, chili powder, cumin, oregano, and smoked paprika. Season with salt and pepper to taste.

4. Bring the chili to a simmer and let it cook for 20•25 minutes, stirring occasionally, until the vegetables are tender and the flavors have melded.

5. Serve the vegetable and bean chili hot, garnished with chopped cilantro if desired. Enjoy!

This hearty, vegetarian chili is packed with fiber, protein, and delicious spices. It's a great meatless main dish or side.

64. Turkey and Avocado Salad

Ingredient:

- 2 cups cooked turkey breast, diced
- 1 avocado, diced
- 1/2 cup diced celery
- 1/4 cup diced red onion
- 2 tbsp plain Greek yogurt
- 1 tbsp Dijon mustard
- 1 tbsp lemon juice
- Salt and pepper to taste
- Mixed greens or lettuce leaves, for serving

Instructions:

1. In a medium bowl, combine the diced cooked turkey, diced avocado, diced celery, and diced red onion.

2. In a small bowl, whisk together the Greek yogurt, Dijon mustard, and lemon juice. Season with salt and pepper.

3. Pour the yogurt dressing over the turkey and avocado mixture and gently toss to coat.

4. Serve the turkey and avocado salad on a bed of mixed greens or lettuce leaves.

This turkey and avocado salad makes a delicious and nutritious meal or snack. The creamy avocado pairs perfectly with the lean turkey, while the crunchy celery and onion add great texture.

The yogurt•based dressing provides a tangy, creamy coating without the extra calories and fat of mayonnaise. You can adjust the amount of dressing to your preference.

This salad is a great way to use up leftover turkey. It's also easy to make ahead and enjoy throughout the week. Enjoy this healthy and flavorful turkey and avocado creation!

65. Baked Chicken Parmesan with Whole Wheat Pasta

Ingredient:

• 4 boneless, skinless chicken breasts
• 1 cup whole wheat breadcrumbs
• 1/2 cup grated Parmesan cheese
• 1 tsp dried oregano
• 1/2 tsp garlic powder
• Salt and pepper to taste
• 1 egg, beaten
• 8 oz whole wheat pasta
• 1 jar (24 oz) marinara sauce
• 1 cup shredded part•skim mozzarella cheese

Instructions:

1. Preheat oven to 400°F. Grease a 9x13 inch baking dish.

2. Pound the chicken breasts to an even thickness, about 1/2 inch thick.

3. In a shallow bowl, combine the breadcrumbs, Parmesan, oregano, garlic powder, salt and pepper.

4. Dip the chicken breasts in the beaten egg, then coat them evenly with the breadcrumb mixture.

5. Place the breaded chicken in the prepared baking dish.

6. Bake for 20•25 minutes, until the chicken is cooked through and the breading is golden brown.

7. Meanwhile, cook the whole wheat pasta according to package instructions. Drain and set aside.

8. Pour the marinara sauce over the baked chicken. Top with the shredded mozzarella cheese.

9. Return the dish to the oven and bake for an additional 10 minutes, until the cheese is melted. Serve the baked chicken parmesan over the cooked whole wheat pasta.

This healthier version of chicken parmesan uses whole wheat breadcrumbs and pasta for added fiber and nutrients. The baked chicken is crispy and flavorful, and pairs perfectly with the classic marinara and melty cheese. Enjoy!

66. Veggie and Hummus Pita

Ingredient:

• 4 whole wheat pita breads, halved
• 1 cup hummus
• 1 cup sliced cucumber
• 1 cup shredded carrots
• 1 cup cherry tomatoes, halved
• 1/2 cup sliced red onion
• 1/4 cup crumbled feta cheese (optional)
• Salt and pepper to taste

Instructions:

1. Spread about 2•3 tablespoons of hummus inside each pita half.

2. Arrange the sliced cucumber, shredded carrots, cherry tomatoes, and red onion slices inside the pita halves.

3. Sprinkle the crumbled feta cheese over the top, if using.

4. Season with a pinch of salt and pepper.

5. Serve the veggie and hummus pitas immediately.

Tips:
• Use your favorite flavor of hummus, such as classic, roasted red pepper, or garlic.
• Feel free to swap in other fresh veggies like bell peppers, sprouts, or avocado.
• For extra protein, add a few slices of grilled chicken or chickpeas.
• Serve with a side salad or fresh fruit for a complete and satisfying meal.

This vegetarian pita pocket is a quick, easy, and nutritious lunch or snack. The combination of creamy hummus and crunchy fresh veggies makes it a delicious and filling option.

67. Spinach and Feta Stuffed Chicken

Ingredient:

• 4 boneless, skinless chicken breasts
• 4 oz crumbled feta cheese
• 1 cup fresh spinach, chopped
• 2 cloves garlic, minced
• 1 tbsp olive oil
• Salt and pepper to taste

For the Sauce:
• 1 cup chicken broth
• 2 tbsp lemon juice
• 1 tsp dried oregano
• 1/4 tsp red pepper flakes (optional)

Instructions:

1. Preheat oven to 375°F.

2. In a medium bowl, mix together the feta cheese, spinach, garlic, and a pinch of salt and pepper.

3. Slice the chicken breasts horizontally to create a pocket. Stuff each chicken breast with the spinach and feta mixture.

4. Heat the olive oil in a large oven•safe skillet over medium•high heat. Add the stuffed chicken breasts and sear for 2•3 minutes per side until golden brown.

5. Transfer the skillet to the preheated oven and bake for 20•25 minutes, until the chicken is cooked through and the internal temperature reaches 165°F.

6. While the chicken is baking, make the sauce. In a small saucepan, combine the chicken broth, lemon juice, oregano, and red pepper flakes (if using). Bring to a simmer and cook for 5 minutes.

7. Remove the chicken from the oven and transfer to a serving plate. Drizzle the warm lemon•oregano sauce over the top.

Serve the spinach and feta stuffed chicken immediately, garnished with extra fresh spinach if desired. Enjoy!

68. Quinoa and Veggie Stuffed Peppers

Ingredient:
• 6 bell peppers, halved and seeded
• 1 cup cooked quinoa
• 1 cup diced zucchini
• 1 cup diced tomatoes
• 1/2 cup diced onion
• 2 cloves garlic, minced
• 1/2 cup crumbled feta cheese
• 2 tbsp chopped fresh basil
• 1 tsp dried oregano
• Salt and pepper to taste
• 1/4 cup shredded mozzarella cheese (optional)

Instructions:

1. Preheat oven to 375°F.

2. Arrange the bell pepper halves in a baking dish or on a rimmed baking sheet.

3. In a large bowl, combine the cooked quinoa, zucchini, tomatoes, onion, garlic, feta cheese, basil, oregano, salt, and pepper. Mix well.

4. Spoon the quinoa and veggie mixture evenly into the bell pepper halves.

5. If using, sprinkle the shredded mozzarella cheese over the top of the stuffed peppers.

6. Bake for 25•30 minutes, until the peppers are tender and the filling is hot.

7. Serve the quinoa and veggie stuffed peppers warm.

Variations:
• Use different colored bell peppers for a colorful presentation.
• Add cooked ground turkey or chicken for extra protein.
• Swap in different veggies like spinach, mushrooms, or corn.
• Top with a drizzle of balsamic glaze or pesto.

These healthy and flavorful stuffed peppers make a great main dish or side. The quinoa and veggie filling is both nutritious and delicious.

69. Grilled Shrimp Salad

Ingredient:

- 1 lb large shrimp, peeled and deveined
- 2 tbsp olive oil
- 1 tsp lemon pepper seasoning
- 6 cups mixed greens (such as spinach, arugula, romaine)
- 1 cup cherry tomatoes, halved
- 1/2 cucumber, sliced
- 1/4 red onion, thinly sliced
- 2 tbsp crumbled feta cheese
- 2 tbsp balsamic vinaigrette

Instructions:

1. Preheat grill or grill pan to medium•high heat.

2. In a medium bowl, toss the shrimp with the olive oil and lemon pepper seasoning.

3. Grill the seasoned shrimp for 2•3 minutes per side, until opaque and cooked through. Remove from heat and set aside.

4. In a large salad bowl, combine the mixed greens, halved cherry tomatoes, cucumber slices, and red onion slices.

5. Top the salad with the grilled shrimp and crumbled feta cheese.

6. Drizzle the balsamic vinaigrette over the top and toss gently to coat.

7. Serve the grilled shrimp salad immediately.

The juicy, flavorful grilled shrimp is the star of this fresh and healthy salad. The combination of crisp greens, juicy tomatoes, crunchy cucumber, and tangy feta creates a delightful balance of textures and flavors.

You can use any type of mixed greens you prefer. The balsamic vinaigrette complements the shrimp and vegetables perfectly.

This grilled shrimp salad makes a light and satisfying main dish. Enjoy!

70. Turkey and Sweet Potato Skillet

Ingredient:

- 1 lb ground turkey
- 2 medium sweet potatoes, peeled and diced
- 1 onion, diced
- 2 cloves garlic, minced
- 1 tsp chili powder
- 1 tsp ground cumin
- 1/2 tsp smoked paprika
- Salt and pepper to taste
- 1 cup low•sodium chicken or vegetable broth
- 1 (15 oz) can black beans, drained and rinsed
- 2 cups baby spinach
- Chopped cilantro for garnish (optional)

Instructions:

1. In a large skillet or cast•iron pan, cook the ground turkey over medium•high heat, breaking it up with a wooden spoon, until browned and cooked through, about 5•7 minutes. Transfer the cooked turkey to a plate.

2. Add the diced sweet potatoes, onion, and garlic to the same skillet. Sauté for 5•7 minutes, until the vegetables start to soften.

3. Stir in the chili powder, cumin, smoked paprika, and a pinch of salt and pepper. Cook for 1 minute to toast the spices.

4. Pour in the broth and scrape up any browned bits from the bottom of the pan. Bring the mixture to a simmer.

5. Reduce the heat to medium•low, cover the skillet, and cook for 10•12 minutes, until the sweet potatoes are tender.

6. Uncover the skillet and stir in the cooked turkey, black beans, and baby spinach. Cook for 2•3 minutes, until the spinach is wilted.

7. Taste and adjust seasoning with additional salt and pepper as needed. Serve the turkey and sweet potato skillet warm, garnished with chopped cilantro if desired.

This one•pan meal is a delicious and nutritious option for a quick weeknight dinner. The combination of lean turkey, sweet potatoes, and black beans makes it a filling and satisfying dish.

71. Greek Yogurt and Berry Parfait

Ingredient:
• 2 cups plain Greek yogurt
• 1 cup fresh berries (such as blueberries, raspberries, or strawberries)
• 2 tbsp honey
• 1/4 cup granola or toasted nuts

Instructions:

1. In a parfait glass or small bowl, layer half of the Greek yogurt.

2. Top the yogurt with half of the fresh berries.

3. Drizzle 1 tbsp of honey over the berries.

4. Repeat the layers, starting with the remaining yogurt, then the remaining berries, and finishing with the last 1 tbsp of honey.

5. Top the parfait with the granola or toasted nuts.

6. Serve chilled.

Variations:
• Use a variety of fresh or frozen berries, such as blackberries, strawberries, raspberries, and blueberries.
• Substitute the honey with maple syrup or agave nectar.
• Add a sprinkle of cinnamon or vanilla extract to the yogurt.
• Use low•fat or non•fat Greek yogurt to make it even healthier.
• Layer the parfait in a mason jar or wine glass for a fun presentation.

This Greek yogurt and berry parfait is a delicious and nutritious breakfast, snack, or dessert. The creamy yogurt, sweet berries, and crunchy granola or nuts make it a satisfying and balanced treat.

72. Chicken and Vegetable Curry

Ingredient:

- 1 lb boneless, skinless chicken breasts, cut into 1•inch pieces
- 2 tbsp olive oil
- 1 onion, diced
- 3 cloves garlic, minced
- 1 tbsp grated fresh ginger
- 2 tsp curry powder
- 1 tsp ground cumin
- 1 tsp ground coriander
- 1/2 tsp cayenne pepper (optional)
- 1 cup diced carrots
- 1 cup diced cauliflower florets
- 1 cup diced zucchini
- 1 cup diced tomatoes
- 1 cup low•sodium chicken broth
- 1 cup coconut milk
- Salt and pepper to taste
- Chopped cilantro for garnish

Instructions:

1. In a large skillet or Dutch oven, heat the olive oil over medium•high heat. Add the chicken and cook for 3•4 minutes, until lightly browned. Transfer the chicken to a plate.

2. Add the onion to the skillet and sauté for 5 minutes until translucent. Add the garlic and ginger and cook for 1 minute, until fragrant.

3. Stir in the curry powder, cumin, coriander, and cayenne (if using). Cook for 1 minute to toast the spices.

4. Add the carrots, cauliflower, zucchini, and tomatoes to the skillet. Pour in the chicken broth and coconut milk. Bring the mixture to a simmer.

5. Return the cooked chicken to the skillet and simmer for 15•20 minutes, until the vegetables are tender and the chicken is cooked through.

6. Season the curry with salt and pepper to taste. Serve the chicken and vegetable curry over basmati rice, garnished with chopped cilantro.

73. Baked Cod with Quinoa and Spinach

Ingredient:

- 4 (6 oz) cod fillets
- 1 cup cooked quinoa
- 2 cups baby spinach, chopped
- 2 tbsp olive oil
- 2 tbsp lemon juice
- 2 cloves garlic, minced
- 1 tsp dried oregano
- Salt and pepper to taste
- Lemon wedges for serving

Instructions:

1. Preheat the oven to 400°F. Lightly grease a baking dish or line with parchment paper.

2. In a medium bowl, combine the cooked quinoa, chopped spinach, 1 tbsp of the olive oil, lemon juice, garlic, and oregano. Season with salt and pepper.

3. Place the cod fillets in the prepared baking dish. Drizzle the remaining 1 tbsp of olive oil over the top of the fish and season with salt and pepper.

4. Spoon the quinoa and spinach mixture over the top of the cod, spreading it out evenly.

5. Bake for 15•18 minutes, until the cod is opaque and flakes easily with a fork.

6. Serve the baked cod immediately, with lemon wedges on the side.

Variations:
- Use other types of white fish like tilapia or halibut.
- Add diced tomatoes, olives, or feta cheese to the quinoa mixture.
- Sprinkle the top with breadcrumbs or Parmesan cheese for extra crunch.
- Serve with roasted vegetables or a fresh salad on the side.

This baked cod with quinoa and spinach is a healthy, flavorful, and easy•to•make meal. The tender fish, nutty quinoa, and fresh spinach make it a nutritious and delicious dinner option.

74. Veggie and Cheese Omelet

Ingredient:

- 3 eggs
- 2 tbsp milk
- 1 tbsp butter
- 1/4 cup diced bell pepper
- 1/4 cup diced onion
- 1/4 cup sliced mushrooms
- 2 tbsp shredded cheddar cheese
- Salt and pepper to taste

Instructions:

1. In a small bowl, whisk together the eggs and milk. Season with a pinch of salt and pepper.

2. Melt the butter in a nonstick skillet over medium heat.

3. Pour the egg mixture into the skillet and let it sit for 20•30 seconds to set the bottom.

4. Using a spatula, gently push the cooked egg from the edges into the center, tilting the pan to allow the uncooked egg to flow to the edges.

5. When the eggs are mostly set but still a bit wet on top, sprinkle the diced bell pepper, onion, and mushrooms over half of the omelet.

6. Fold the other half of the omelet over the veggie•filled half.

7. Sprinkle the shredded cheddar cheese over the top.

8. Cook for 1•2 minutes more, until the cheese is melted and the omelet is cooked through. Slide the veggie and cheese omelet onto a plate and serve immediately.

Variations:
- Use different veggies like spinach, tomatoes, or zucchini.
- Try different cheese varieties like feta, goat cheese, or Swiss.
- Add a dash of hot sauce or salsa for extra flavor.

This veggie and cheese omelet is a delicious and nutritious way to start your day. The fluffy eggs, melty cheese, and fresh veggies make it a satisfying breakfast option.

75. Beef and Sweet Potato Stir•Fry

Ingredient:

• 1 lb beef sirloin or flank steak, thinly sliced
• 2 medium sweet potatoes, peeled and cut into 1•inch cubes
• 1 red bell pepper, sliced
• 1 cup broccoli florets
• 2 cloves garlic, minced
• 1 tbsp grated fresh ginger
• 2 tbsp low•sodium soy sauce
• 1 tbsp rice vinegar
• 1 tsp sesame oil
• 1 tsp cornstarch
• 2 tbsp vegetable oil
• Salt and pepper to taste
• Chopped green onions for garnish (optional)

Instructions:

1. In a small bowl, whisk together the soy sauce, rice vinegar, sesame oil, and cornstarch. Set aside.

2. Heat the vegetable oil in a large skillet or wok over high heat. Add the beef and stir•fry for 2•3 minutes until browned. Transfer the beef to a plate.

3. Add the sweet potato cubes to the skillet and stir•fry for 5•7 minutes, until starting to soften.

4. Add the bell pepper, broccoli, garlic, and ginger to the skillet. Stir•fry for 3•4 minutes.

5. Return the beef to the skillet and pour in the soy sauce mixture. Toss everything together and cook for 2•3 minutes, until the sauce has thickened and the vegetables are tender•crisp.

6. Season the stir•fry with salt and pepper to taste. Serve the beef and sweet potato stir•fry immediately, garnished with chopped green onions if desired. Enjoy over steamed rice or noodles.

This beef and sweet potato stir•fry is a quick, healthy, and flavorful meal. The combination of tender beef, sweet potatoes, and crisp vegetables makes it a satisfying one•pan dish.

76. Grilled Chicken and Veggie Kabobs

Ingredient:
• 1 lb boneless, skinless chicken breasts, cut into 1•inch cubes
• 1 red bell pepper, cut into 1•inch pieces
• 1 zucchini, cut into 1•inch slices
• 1 red onion, cut into 1•inch pieces
• 8 oz mushrooms, halved
• 2 tbsp olive oil
• 2 tbsp lemon juice
• 1 tsp dried oregano
• 1 tsp garlic powder
• Salt and pepper to taste
• Wooden or metal skewers

Instructions:
1. In a large bowl, combine the cubed chicken, bell pepper, zucchini, onion, and mushrooms.

2. In a small bowl, whisk together the olive oil, lemon juice, oregano, garlic powder, salt, and pepper.

3. Pour the marinade over the chicken and vegetables and toss to coat everything evenly.

4. Thread the marinated chicken and vegetables onto the skewers, alternating the ingredients.

5. Preheat your grill to medium•high heat.

6. Grill the kabobs for 12•15 minutes, turning occasionally, until the chicken is cooked through and the vegetables are tender. Serve the grilled chicken and veggie kabobs immediately.

Variations:
• Use different vegetables like cherry tomatoes, pineapple chunks, or eggplant.
• Marinate the kabobs in a teriyaki or balsamic vinaigrette instead.
• Add cubes of halloumi or feta cheese to the skewers.
• Serve the kabobs with a side of rice, quinoa, or a fresh salad.

These grilled chicken and veggie kabobs are a fun, healthy, and delicious summer meal. The combination of juicy chicken and roasted vegetables makes them a crowd•pleasing option for backyard barbecues or weeknight dinners.

77. Tuna and White Bean Salad

Ingredient:

• 2 (5 oz) cans tuna, drained
• 1 (15 oz) can white beans, drained and rinsed
• 1/2 cup diced celery
• 1/4 cup diced red onion
• 2 tbsp chopped fresh parsley
• 2 tbsp lemon juice
• 2 tbsp olive oil
• 1 tsp Dijon mustard
• Salt and pepper to taste

Instructions:

1. In a medium bowl, gently flake the tuna with a fork.

2. Add the drained and rinsed white beans, diced celery, diced red onion, and chopped parsley. Stir to combine.

3. In a small bowl, whisk together the lemon juice, olive oil, and Dijon mustard. Season with salt and pepper.

4. Pour the dressing over the tuna and bean mixture and toss gently to coat.

5. Serve the tuna and white bean salad chilled or at room temperature. It can be served on its own, over a bed of greens, or stuffed into tomatoes or avocado halves.

Variations:
• Use chickpeas or kidney beans instead of white beans.
• Add diced cucumber, bell pepper, or cherry tomatoes.
• Sprinkle with crumbled feta or shredded cheddar cheese.
• Use fresh herbs like basil, dill, or chives.
• For extra flavor, add a pinch of red pepper flakes or dried oregano.

This tuna and white bean salad is a quick, easy, and nutritious lunch or light dinner option. The combination of protein•rich tuna and fiber•filled beans makes it a satisfying and wholesome meal.

78. Sweet Potato and Black Bean Enchiladas

Ingredient:

- 2 medium sweet potatoes, peeled and diced
- 1 (15 oz) can black beans, drained and rinsed
- 1 cup diced onion
- 2 cloves garlic, minced
- 1 tsp ground cumin
- 1 tsp chili powder
- Salt and pepper to taste
- 8 whole wheat tortillas
- 1 (15 oz) can enchilada sauce
- 1 cup shredded Mexican cheese blend

Instructions:

1. Preheat the oven to 375°F. Grease a 9x13 inch baking dish.

2. In a large skillet, sauté the diced sweet potatoes over medium heat for 8•10 minutes, until tender.

3. Add the black beans, diced onion, and minced garlic to the skillet. Cook for 2•3 minutes, until the onion is translucent.

4. Stir in the cumin, chili powder, and season with salt and pepper to taste.

5. Spread 1/4 cup of the sweet potato and black bean mixture onto each tortilla. Roll up the tortillas and place seam•side down in the prepared baking dish.

6. Pour the enchilada sauce evenly over the top of the enchiladas. Sprinkle the shredded cheese over the sauce.

7. Bake for 20•25 minutes, until the cheese is melted and bubbly.Serve the sweet potato and black bean enchiladas warm, garnished with chopped cilantro or green onions if desired.

These sweet potato and black bean enchiladas are a delicious and nutritious meatless main dish. The combination of roasted sweet potatoes, protein•packed beans, and warm spices makes for a satisfying and flavorful meal.

79. Cottage Cheese with Sliced Peaches

Ingredient:

• 1 cup low•fat or non•fat cottage cheese
• 1 medium peach, sliced
• 1 tsp honey (optional)
• Cinnamon for garnish (optional)

Instructions:

1. Scoop the cottage cheese into a bowl or serving dish.

2. Arrange the sliced peaches on top of the cottage cheese.

3. If desired, drizzle the honey over the peaches and cottage cheese.

4. Sprinkle a light dusting of cinnamon over the top as a garnish.

That's it! This healthy snack or light meal comes together in just a few minutes.

Variations:
• Use nectarines, plums, or other stone fruits instead of peaches.
• Top with a sprinkle of granola or chopped nuts for added crunch.
• Swap the honey for a drizzle of maple syrup or agave nectar.
• Add a handful of fresh berries like blueberries or raspberries.
• Use flavored cottage cheese like pineapple or herb•garlic.

The combination of creamy cottage cheese and sweet, juicy peaches makes for a refreshing and nutritious snack or breakfast. The cottage cheese provides protein, while the peaches offer fiber, vitamins, and natural sweetness. It's a simple but satisfying way to enjoy seasonal produce.

80. Chicken and Avocado Wrap

Ingredient:

• 2 cups shredded cooked chicken
• 1 avocado, sliced
• 1/2 cup diced tomatoes
• 1/4 cup diced red onion
• 2 tbsp chopped fresh cilantro
• 2 tbsp lime juice
• 1 tsp olive oil
• Salt and pepper to taste
• 4 whole wheat tortillas or wraps

Instructions:

1. In a medium bowl, combine the shredded chicken, sliced avocado, diced tomatoes, diced red onion, and chopped cilantro.

2. Drizzle the lime juice and olive oil over the mixture and gently toss to coat.

3. Season the chicken and avocado mixture with salt and pepper to taste.

4. Lay the tortillas or wraps out on a flat surface. Divide the chicken and avocado mixture evenly among the wraps, placing it in the center.

5. Fold the bottom of the wrap up over the filling, then fold in the sides and continue rolling up tightly to enclose the filling.

6. Serve the chicken and avocado wraps immediately, or wrap them in parchment paper or foil to enjoy later.

Variations:
• Add shredded lettuce, diced cucumber, or crumbled feta cheese.
• Use grilled or blackened chicken for extra flavor.
• Swap the tortillas for spinach or whole grain wraps.
• Drizzle with a creamy chipotle or ranch dressing.
• Serve the wraps with a side of salsa or guacamole for dipping.

These chicken and avocado wraps make a delicious and portable lunch or snack. The creamy avocado, juicy chicken, and fresh veggies create a satisfying and nutritious meal.

81. Lentil and Vegetable Curry

Ingredient:

- 1 cup dried brown or green lentils, rinsed
- 1 tbsp olive oil
- 1 onion, diced
- 3 cloves garlic, minced
- 1 tbsp grated fresh ginger
- 2 tsp curry powder
- 1 tsp ground cumin
- 1 tsp ground coriander
- 1/2 tsp cayenne pepper (optional)
- 1 cup diced carrots
- 1 cup diced cauliflower florets
- 1 cup diced potatoes
- 1 (14 oz) can diced tomatoes
- 1 (13.5 oz) can coconut milk
- 1 cup vegetable broth
- Salt and pepper to taste
- Chopped cilantro for garnish

Instructions:

1. In a large pot, cover the lentils with water and bring to a boil. Reduce heat and simmer for 15•20 minutes, until lentils are tender. Drain and set aside.

2. In the same pot, heat the olive oil over medium heat. Add the onion and sauté for 5 minutes until translucent.

3. Stir in the garlic, ginger, curry powder, cumin, coriander, and cayenne (if using). Cook for 1 minute to toast the spices.

4. Add the carrots, cauliflower, and potatoes to the pot. Pour in the diced tomatoes, coconut milk, and vegetable broth. Bring the mixture to a simmer.

5. Reduce heat to medium•low and let the curry simmer for 20•25 minutes, until the vegetables are tender.

6. Stir the cooked lentils into the curry. Season with salt and pepper to taste.

7. Serve the lentil and vegetable curry warm, garnished with chopped cilantro. Enjoy over basmati rice or with naan bread.

This hearty and flavorful lentil and vegetable curry is a delicious meatless main dish. The combination of spices, creamy coconut milk, and tender vegetables makes it a comforting and satisfying meal.

82. Turkey and Quinoa Meatloaf

Ingredient:

• 1 lb ground turkey
• 1 cup cooked quinoa
• 1 egg, beaten
• 1/2 cup diced onion
• 1/2 cup diced bell pepper
• 2 cloves garlic, minced
• 1 tsp dried oregano
• 1 tsp dried basil
• 1/2 tsp salt
• 1/4 tsp black pepper
• 1/4 cup ketchup or tomato sauce

Instructions:

1. Preheat the oven to 375°F. Grease a 9x5 inch loaf pan.

2. In a large bowl, combine the ground turkey, cooked quinoa, beaten egg, diced onion, diced bell pepper, minced garlic, oregano, basil, salt, and pepper. Mix well until all the ingredients are evenly distributed.

3. Transfer the turkey and quinoa mixture to the prepared loaf pan, pressing it down firmly.

4. Spread the ketchup or tomato sauce evenly over the top of the meatloaf.

5. Bake for 50•60 minutes, until the internal temperature reaches 165°F. Let the meatloaf rest for 5•10 minutes before slicing and serving.

Variations:
• Use a combination of ground turkey and ground beef or pork.
• Add shredded carrots, spinach, or mushrooms to the meatloaf mixture.
• Top the meatloaf with barbecue sauce, teriyaki glaze, or a brown sugar•mustard topping.
• Serve the turkey and quinoa meatloaf with mashed potatoes, roasted vegetables, or a fresh salad.

This turkey and quinoa meatloaf is a healthier twist on a classic comfort food. The quinoa adds fiber, protein, and a nice texture, while the turkey keeps the meatloaf lean and flavorful. It's a delicious and nutritious main dish the whole family will enjoy.

83. Greek Salad with Tuna

Ingredient:

• 1 head romaine lettuce, chopped
• 1 cup cherry tomatoes, halved
• 1 cucumber, diced
• 1/2 red onion, thinly sliced
• 1 (5 oz) can tuna, drained
• 1/2 cup pitted kalamata olives, halved
• 1/2 cup crumbled feta cheese
• 2 tbsp olive oil
• 1 tbsp red wine vinegar
• 1 tsp dried oregano
• Salt and pepper to taste

Instructions:

1. In a large salad bowl, combine the chopped romaine lettuce, cherry tomatoes, diced cucumber, and sliced red onion.

2. Flake the drained tuna over the top of the salad.

3. Sprinkle the kalamata olives and crumbled feta cheese over the salad.

4. In a small bowl, whisk together the olive oil, red wine vinegar, and dried oregano. Season the dressing with salt and pepper.

5. Drizzle the dressing over the salad and toss gently to coat.

6. Serve the Greek salad with tuna immediately.

Variations:
• Add other veggies like bell peppers, artichoke hearts, or pepperoncini.
• Use canned chickpeas or white beans instead of tuna for a vegetarian option.
• Swap the feta for crumbled goat cheese or shredded mozzarella.
• Garnish with fresh herbs like parsley, basil, or dill.
• Serve the salad with pita bread or crusty bread on the side.

This Greek salad with tuna is a light, refreshing, and protein•packed meal. The combination of crisp greens, juicy tomatoes, briny olives, and flavorful tuna makes it a delicious and nutritious option.

84. Broccoli and Cheese Stuffed Chicken

Ingredient:

• 4 boneless, skinless chicken breasts
• 1 cup chopped broccoli florets
• 1/2 cup shredded cheddar cheese
• 2 tbsp cream cheese, softened
• 1 tsp dried parsley
• 1/2 tsp garlic powder
• Salt and pepper to taste
• 1 tbsp olive oil

Instructions:

1. Preheat the oven to 375°F. Grease a baking dish or line it with parchment paper.

2. In a medium bowl, mix together the chopped broccoli, shredded cheddar cheese, cream cheese, dried parsley, garlic powder, and a pinch of salt and pepper.

3. Slice each chicken breast horizontally to create a pocket, being careful not to cut all the way through.

4. Stuff the broccoli and cheese mixture evenly into the pockets of the chicken breasts.

5. Heat the olive oil in a large oven•safe skillet over medium•high heat. Add the stuffed chicken breasts and sear for 2•3 minutes per side until golden brown.

6. Transfer the skillet to the preheated oven and bake for 20•25 minutes, until the chicken is cooked through and the internal temperature reaches 165°F.

7. Remove the broccoli and cheese stuffed chicken from the oven and let it rest for 5 minutes before serving.

Variations:
• Use a different type of cheese, such as mozzarella or Parmesan.
• Add diced bacon or chopped spinach to the filling.
• Sprinkle the top of the chicken with breadcrumbs or crushed crackers for extra crunch.
• Serve the stuffed chicken with a side of roasted vegetables or a fresh salad.

This broccoli and cheese stuffed chicken is a delicious and easy•to•make main dish. The creamy, cheesy filling complements the juicy chicken perfectly, making it a satisfying and flavorful meal.

85. Shrimp and Quinoa Stir•Fry

Ingredient:

- 1 cup uncooked quinoa, rinsed
- 1 lb shrimp, peeled and deveined
- 2 tbsp sesame oil
- 2 cloves garlic, minced
- 1 tbsp grated fresh ginger
- 1 red bell pepper, sliced
- 1 cup broccoli florets
- 2 cups baby spinach
- 2 tbsp low•sodium soy sauce
- 1 tbsp rice vinegar
- 1 tsp sesame seeds (optional)
- Salt and pepper to taste

Instructions:

1. Cook the quinoa according to package instructions. Fluff with a fork and set aside.

2. In a large skillet or wok, heat the sesame oil over medium•high heat. Add the shrimp and sauté for 2•3 minutes until they start to turn pink.

3. Add the minced garlic and grated ginger to the skillet. Cook for 1 minute, until fragrant.

4. Stir in the sliced red bell pepper and broccoli florets. Sauté for 3•4 minutes, until the vegetables are tender•crisp.

5. Add the cooked quinoa, baby spinach, soy sauce, and rice vinegar to the skillet. Toss everything together and cook for 2•3 minutes, until the spinach is wilted.

6. Season the shrimp and quinoa stir•fry with salt and pepper to taste.

7. Serve the stir•fry warm, garnished with sesame seeds if desired.

This shrimp and quinoa stir•fry is a quick, healthy, and delicious meal. The combination of protein•rich shrimp, nutrient•dense quinoa, and fresh vegetables makes it a satisfying and well•balanced dish.

86. Apple and Peanut Butter Sandwich

Ingredient:

• 2 slices whole wheat bread
• 2 tbsp creamy peanut butter
• 1 medium apple, thinly sliced
• 1 tsp honey (optional)
• Cinnamon (optional)

Instructions:

1. Spread the peanut butter evenly on one slice of bread.

2. Arrange the apple slices in a single layer on top of the peanut butter.

3. Drizzle the honey over the apple slices, if using.

4. Sprinkle a light dusting of cinnamon over the apples, if desired.

5. Top with the second slice of bread to create a sandwich.

6. Cut the sandwich in half and serve immediately.

Variations:
• Use almond butter or cashew butter instead of peanut butter.
• Add a sprinkle of granola or crushed nuts for extra crunch.
• Swap the apple for sliced banana or pear.
• Toast the bread before assembling the sandwich.
• Serve the sandwich with a side of Greek yogurt or a piece of fruit.

This apple and peanut butter sandwich is a simple, healthy, and delicious snack or light meal. The combination of creamy peanut butter, crisp apple slices, and a touch of sweetness from the honey makes it a satisfying and nutritious option. It's a great way to incorporate more fruit into your day.

87. Grilled Vegetable and Cheese Quesadilla

Ingredient:

- 1 zucchini, sliced into 1/4·inch rounds
- 1 red bell pepper, sliced into strips
- 1 onion, sliced into rings
- 1 tbsp olive oil
- Salt and pepper to taste
- 4 whole wheat tortillas
- 1 cup shredded Mexican cheese blend
- 2 tbsp chopped fresh cilantro (optional)

Instructions:

1. Preheat a grill or grill pan to medium·high heat.

2. In a large bowl, toss the sliced zucchini, bell pepper, and onion with the olive oil. Season with salt and pepper.

3. Grill the vegetables for 3·5 minutes per side, until tender and slightly charred.

4. Remove the grilled vegetables from the grill and let them cool slightly.

5. Lay the tortillas out on a flat surface. Sprinkle half of each tortilla with the shredded cheese, leaving a small border.

6. Top the cheese with the grilled vegetables, distributing them evenly. Sprinkle with the chopped cilantro, if using.

7. Fold the empty half of the tortilla over the filled half to create a half·moon shape.

8. Carefully transfer the quesadillas to the grill or grill pan. Cook for 2·3 minutes per side, until the tortilla is lightly golden and the cheese is melted.

9. Remove the grilled vegetable and cheese quesadillas from the grill and cut each one in half to serve.

This grilled vegetable and cheese quesadilla is a delicious and healthy twist on a classic Mexican dish. The combination of tender grilled veggies and melted cheese makes it a satisfying and flavorful meal or snack.

88. Chicken and Brown Rice Casserole

Ingredient:

• 1 cup uncooked brown rice
• 1 lb boneless, skinless chicken breasts, cubed
• 1 onion, diced
• 2 cloves garlic, minced
• 1 cup sliced mushrooms
• 1 cup frozen peas
• 1 (10.5 oz) can reduced•sodium cream of mushroom soup
• 1/2 cup low•sodium chicken broth
• 1/2 tsp dried thyme
• 1/2 tsp dried rosemary
• Salt and pepper to taste
• 1/2 cup shredded cheddar cheese

Instructions:

1. Preheat the oven to 375°F. Grease a 9x13 inch baking dish.

2. Cook the brown rice according to package instructions. Set aside.

3. In a large skillet, sauté the cubed chicken over medium•high heat until browned, about 5•7 minutes. Transfer the chicken to a plate.

4. In the same skillet, sauté the diced onion for 3•4 minutes until translucent. Add the minced garlic and sliced mushrooms, and cook for 2 more minutes.

5. Stir the cooked chicken, cooked brown rice, frozen peas, cream of mushroom soup, chicken broth, thyme, rosemary, salt, and pepper into the skillet with the vegetables. Mix well.

6. Transfer the chicken and rice mixture to the prepared baking dish. Sprinkle the shredded cheddar cheese evenly over the top.

7. Bake the casserole for 25•30 minutes, until the cheese is melted and bubbly.

8. Let the casserole cool for 5 minutes before serving.

This chicken and brown rice casserole is a comforting and nutritious one•dish meal. The combination of tender chicken, nutty brown rice, and a creamy sauce makes it a satisfying and family•friendly option.

89. Spaghetti Squash with Pesto

Ingredient:

• 1 medium spaghetti squash, halved lengthwise and seeded
• 2 tbsp olive oil
• Salt and pepper to taste
• 1/2 cup basil pesto (store•bought or homemade)
• 2 tbsp toasted pine nuts (optional)
• Grated Parmesan cheese for serving (optional)

Instructions:

1. Preheat the oven to 400°F. Line a baking sheet with parchment paper.

2. Place the spaghetti squash halves cut•side up on the prepared baking sheet. Drizzle the squash with the olive oil and season with salt and pepper.

3. Roast the spaghetti squash for 40•50 minutes, until tender when pierced with a fork.

4. Remove the squash from the oven and let it cool slightly. Using a fork, gently scrape the flesh of the squash to create long, spaghetti•like strands.

5. Transfer the spaghetti squash strands to a serving bowl. Toss the squash with the basil pesto until evenly coated.

6. Top the pesto spaghetti squash with the toasted pine nuts, if using, and a sprinkle of grated Parmesan cheese.

7. Serve the spaghetti squash with pesto warm.

Variations:
• Use a different type of pesto, such as sun•dried tomato or arugula pesto.
• Add sautéed mushrooms, cherry tomatoes, or grilled chicken for extra protein.
• Sprinkle with toasted breadcrumbs or crushed almonds for crunch.
• Serve the spaghetti squash with a side salad or garlic bread.

This spaghetti squash with pesto is a delicious and healthy alternative to traditional pasta. The nutty, herby pesto complements the sweet and tender spaghetti squash perfectly. It's a great way to enjoy a low•carb, veggie•based meal.

90. Grilled Fish Tacos

Ingredient:

• 1 lb white fish fillets (such as tilapia, cod, or halibut)
• 2 tbsp olive oil
• 1 tsp chili powder
• 1 tsp cumin
• 1/2 tsp garlic powder
• Salt and pepper to taste
• 8•10 small corn or flour tortillas
• 1 cup shredded cabbage or coleslaw mix
• 1/2 cup diced tomatoes
• 1/4 cup chopped cilantro
• 1/4 cup crumbled feta or queso fresco
• Lime wedges for serving

For the Chipotle Crema:
• 1/2 cup plain Greek yogurt
• 2 tbsp mayonnaise
• 1 tbsp lime juice
• 1 tsp adobo sauce from canned chipotle peppers
• Salt and pepper to taste

Instructions:

1. In a shallow dish, combine the olive oil, chili powder, cumin, garlic powder, salt, and pepper. Add the fish fillets and turn to coat both sides.

2. Preheat a grill or grill pan to medium•high heat. Grill the fish for 3•4 minutes per side, until cooked through and flaky.

3. In a small bowl, mix together the ingredients for the chipotle crema. Season with salt and pepper to taste.

4. Warm the tortillas according to package instructions.

5. Flake the grilled fish into bite•sized pieces.

6. To assemble the tacos, place some of the fish in the center of each tortilla. Top with shredded cabbage, diced tomatoes, chopped cilantro, and crumbled feta or queso fresco.

7. Drizzle the chipotle crema over the top of the tacos. Serve the grilled fish tacos immediately, with lime wedges on the side.

These grilled fish tacos are a light, fresh, and flavorful meal. The combination of tender fish, crunchy slaw, and creamy chipotle crema makes them a delicious and satisfying option.

91. Cottage Cheese and Berry Smoothie

Ingredient:

• 1 cup low•fat or non•fat cottage cheese
• 1 cup frozen mixed berries (such as strawberries, blueberries, and raspberries)
• 1/2 cup unsweetened almond milk (or milk of your choice)
• 1 tbsp honey (optional)
• 1/2 tsp vanilla extract

Instructions:

1. In a blender, combine the cottage cheese, frozen berries, almond milk, honey (if using), and vanilla extract.

2. Blend the ingredients on high speed until smooth and creamy, about 1•2 minutes.

3. Pour the cottage cheese and berry smoothie into a glass and serve immediately.

Variations:
• Use plain Greek yogurt instead of cottage cheese for a thicker consistency.
• Add a handful of spinach or kale for extra nutrients.
• Swap the berries for other frozen fruit like mango or pineapple.
• Use vanilla•flavored protein powder for a boost of protein.
• Top the smoothie with a sprinkle of granola or chopped nuts.

This cottage cheese and berry smoothie is a delicious and nutritious breakfast or snack option. The cottage cheese provides protein, while the berries and almond milk offer fiber, vitamins, and antioxidants. It's a great way to start your day or refuel after a workout.

The smooth, creamy texture and natural sweetness make this smoothie a satisfying and healthy treat. It's a versatile recipe that can be customized to your taste preferences.

92. Chicken Caesar Wrap

Ingredient:

• 2 cups shredded cooked chicken
• 2 tbsp Caesar dressing
• 2 cups chopped romaine lettuce
• 1/4 cup shredded Parmesan cheese
• 2 tbsp croutons, crushed
• 4 whole wheat tortillas or wraps

Instructions:

1. In a medium bowl, mix together the shredded chicken and Caesar dressing until the chicken is evenly coated.

2. Lay the tortillas or wraps out on a flat surface. Divide the chopped romaine lettuce evenly among the wraps, placing it in the center.

3. Top the lettuce with the Caesar•coated chicken, shredded Parmesan cheese, and crushed croutons.

4. Fold the bottom of the wrap up over the filling, then fold in the sides and continue rolling up tightly to enclose the filling.

5. Serve the chicken Caesar wraps immediately, or wrap them in parchment paper or foil to enjoy later.

Variations:
• Use grilled or blackened chicken for extra flavor.
• Add diced tomatoes, sliced cucumber, or shredded carrots.
• Swap the Parmesan for crumbled feta or shredded cheddar.
• Use a flavored tortilla, such as garlic or spinach.
• Drizzle with a balsamic glaze or hot sauce for extra zing.
• Serve the wraps with a side of Caesar salad or fresh fruit.

This chicken Caesar wrap is a quick, easy, and portable lunch or snack option. The combination of tender chicken, crisp romaine, creamy Caesar dressing, and crunchy Parmesan and croutons makes it a satisfying and flavorful meal.

93. Baked Eggplant Parmesan

Ingredient:

• 2 medium eggplants, sliced into 1/2•inch thick rounds
• 2 eggs, beaten
• 1 cup breadcrumbs
• 1 cup grated Parmesan cheese
• 1 tsp dried oregano
• 1 tsp garlic powder
• 1/2 tsp salt
• 1/4 tsp black pepper
• 2 cups marinara sauce
• 2 cups shredded mozzarella cheese

Instructions:

1. Preheat oven to 400°F. Line a baking sheet with parchment paper.

2. In a shallow bowl, beat the eggs. In another shallow bowl, mix together the breadcrumbs, Parmesan, oregano, garlic powder, salt, and pepper.

3. Dip the eggplant slices into the beaten egg, then coat both sides in the breadcrumb mixture, pressing to adhere. Place the breaded eggplant slices in a single layer on the prepared baking sheet.

4. Bake for 20 minutes, flip the slices, then bake for another 15•20 minutes until golden brown and crispy.

5. Spread 1 cup of the marinara sauce in the bottom of a 9x13 inch baking dish. Arrange the baked eggplant slices in a single layer on top of the sauce. Top with the remaining 1 cup of marinara sauce and the shredded mozzarella cheese.

6. Bake for 15•20 minutes, until the cheese is melted and bubbly.

7. Let stand for 5 minutes before serving.

94. Tuna and Avocado Wrap

Ingredient:

• 1 (5 oz) can tuna, drained
• 1 ripe avocado, diced
• 2 tbsp plain Greek yogurt
• 1 tsp lemon juice
• 1/4 tsp salt
• 1/4 tsp black pepper
• 2 whole wheat tortillas or wraps

Instructions:

1. In a medium bowl, mix together the drained tuna, diced avocado, Greek yogurt, lemon juice, salt, and black pepper until well combined.

2. Lay the tortillas or wraps out flat. Divide the tuna and avocado mixture evenly between the two wraps, spreading it out in a line down the center of each wrap.

3. Fold the bottom of the wrap up over the filling, then fold in the sides and continue rolling up tightly into a wrap.

4. Serve immediately or wrap in parchment paper or foil to enjoy later. The wrap can be refrigerated for up to 2 days.

95. Sweet Potato and Black Bean Burrito

Ingredient:

• 2 medium sweet potatoes, peeled and diced
• 1 tbsp olive oil
• 1 onion, diced
• 2 cloves garlic, minced
• 1 (15 oz) can black beans, drained and rinsed
• 1 tsp ground cumin
• 1 tsp chili powder
• Salt and pepper to taste
• 6 large whole wheat tortillas
• 1 cup shredded cheddar or Monterey Jack cheese
• Chopped cilantro for garnish (optional)

Instructions:

1. Preheat the oven to 400°F. Toss the diced sweet potatoes with the olive oil and spread them out on a baking sheet. Roast for 20•25 minutes, until tender.

2. In a skillet over medium heat, sauté the diced onion for 5 minutes until translucent. Add the minced garlic and cook for 1 minute more.

3. Stir the roasted sweet potatoes and drained black beans into the skillet with the onions and garlic. Season with the cumin, chili powder, salt, and pepper. Cook for 2•3 minutes to heat through.

4. Lay the tortillas out on a flat surface. Spoon the sweet potato and black bean mixture down the center of each tortilla. Top with a sprinkle of shredded cheese.

5. Fold the bottom of the tortilla up over the filling, then fold in the sides and continue rolling up tightly to enclose the filling.

6. Place the burritos seam•side down on a baking sheet. Bake for 10•12 minutes, until the tortillas are lightly golden.

7. Serve the sweet potato and black bean burritos warm, garnished with chopped cilantro if desired.

This sweet potato and black bean burrito is a delicious and nutritious vegetarian meal. The combination of roasted sweet potatoes, protein•packed beans, and warm spices makes it a satisfying and flavorful option.

96. Veggie and Cheese Frittata

Ingredient:

• 8 large eggs
• 1/4 cup milk or unsweetened almond milk
• 1/2 tsp salt
• 1/4 tsp black pepper
• 1 tbsp olive oil
• 1 cup diced bell peppers
• 1 cup diced onions
• 2 cups chopped spinach or kale
• 1 cup shredded cheddar or mozzarella cheese

Instructions:

1. Preheat oven to 375°F.

2. In a medium bowl, whisk together the eggs, milk, salt, and pepper until well combined.

3. Heat the olive oil in a 9•inch oven•safe non•stick skillet over medium heat.

4. Add the diced bell peppers and onions to the skillet. Cook for 3•4 minutes, stirring occasionally, until the vegetables are softened.

5. Add the chopped spinach or kale to the skillet and cook for 1•2 minutes until wilted.

6. Pour the egg mixture over the vegetables in the skillet. Sprinkle the shredded cheese evenly over the top.

7. Transfer the skillet to the preheated oven and bake for 15•20 minutes, until the eggs are set and the top is lightly golden.

8. Remove the frittata from the oven and let it cool for 5 minutes before slicing and serving.

Serve the Veggie and Cheese Frittata warm, either on its own or with a side salad. Enjoy!

97. Chicken and Veggie Skillet

Ingredient:

• 1 lb boneless, skinless chicken breasts, cut into 1•inch cubes
• 2 tbsp olive oil
• 1 cup diced bell peppers
• 1 cup diced onions
• 2 cups chopped broccoli florets
• 1 cup sliced mushrooms
• 2 cloves garlic, minced
• 1 tsp dried oregano
• 1/2 tsp salt
• 1/4 tsp black pepper
• 1/4 cup low•sodium chicken broth

Instructions:

1. Heat the olive oil in a large skillet or sauté pan over medium•high heat.

2. Add the cubed chicken to the skillet and cook for 5•7 minutes, stirring occasionally, until the chicken is lightly browned on all sides. Remove the chicken from the skillet and set aside.

3. Add the diced bell peppers and onions to the same skillet. Cook for 3•4 minutes, stirring occasionally, until the vegetables start to soften.

4. Add the chopped broccoli, sliced mushrooms, and minced garlic to the skillet. Cook for 2•3 minutes, stirring frequently, until the vegetables are tender•crisp.

5. Return the cooked chicken to the skillet. Sprinkle the dried oregano, salt, and black pepper over the top.

6. Pour in the chicken broth and stir to combine. Bring the mixture to a simmer and cook for 2•3 minutes, until the sauce has thickened slightly.

7. Remove the skillet from heat and serve the Chicken and Veggie Skillet immediately, while hot.

This dish can be served on its own or over a bed of cooked quinoa or brown rice. Enjoy your healthy and delicious Chicken and Veggie Skillet!

98. Quinoa and Spinach Salad

Ingredient:

- 1 cup uncooked quinoa, rinsed
- 2 cups vegetable or chicken broth
- 4 cups fresh spinach, chopped
- 1 cup cherry tomatoes, halved
- 1/2 cup cucumber, diced
- 1/4 cup red onion, thinly sliced
- 2 tbsp crumbled feta cheese
- 2 tbsp toasted sliced almonds

Dressing:

- 2 tbsp olive oil
- 1 tbsp lemon juice
- 1 tsp Dijon mustard
- 1 tsp honey
- 1/4 tsp salt
- 1/4 tsp black pepper

Instructions:

1. In a medium saucepan, combine the quinoa and broth. Bring to a boil, then reduce heat to low, cover and simmer for 15•20 minutes until quinoa is cooked and liquid is absorbed. Fluff with a fork and let cool.

2. In a large bowl, combine the cooked quinoa, spinach, tomatoes, cucumber, and red onion.

3. In a small bowl, whisk together the olive oil, lemon juice, Dijon mustard, honey, salt and pepper to make the dressing.

4. Pour the dressing over the quinoa salad and toss gently to coat.

5. Top the salad with the crumbled feta cheese and toasted almonds.

6. Serve immediately or refrigerate until ready to serve.

99. Grilled Steak Salad

Ingredient:

- 1 lb flank steak or skirt steak
- 2 tbsp olive oil
- 1 tsp garlic powder
- 1 tsp dried oregano
- 1/2 tsp salt
- 1/4 tsp black pepper
- 8 cups mixed greens (such as spinach, arugula, and romaine)
- 1 cup cherry tomatoes, halved
- 1/2 cup sliced cucumber
- 1/4 cup thinly sliced red onion
- 2 tbsp crumbled feta cheese
- 2 tbsp balsamic vinaigrette

Instructions:

1. Preheat grill or grill pan to medium·high heat.

2. In a small bowl, combine the olive oil, garlic powder, oregano, salt, and black pepper. Rub the seasoning mixture all over the steak.

3. Grill the steak for 4·6 minutes per side, or until it reaches your desired level of doneness. Transfer the steak to a cutting board and let it rest for 5 minutes.

4. Slice the steak against the grain into thin strips.

5. In a large salad bowl, combine the mixed greens, cherry tomatoes, cucumber, and red onion.

6. Top the salad with the grilled steak strips and crumbled feta cheese.

7. Drizzle the balsamic vinaigrette over the top and toss gently to coat.

8. Serve the Grilled Steak Salad immediately.

100. Hummus and Veggie Plate

Ingredient:

• 1 cup homemade or store•bought hummus
• 1 cup baby carrots
• 1 cup cucumber slices
• 1 cup cherry tomatoes
• 1 cup bell pepper strips (red, yellow, or orange)
• 1 cup broccoli florets
• 1/4 cup roasted unsalted almonds
• 2 tbsp crumbled feta cheese (optional)
• 1 tbsp chopped fresh parsley (optional)

Instructions:

1. Arrange the hummus in the center of a large plate or platter.

2. Arrange the baby carrots, cucumber slices, cherry tomatoes, bell pepper strips, and broccoli florets around the hummus in a decorative pattern.

3. Sprinkle the roasted almonds over the top of the hummus.

4. If desired, sprinkle the crumbled feta cheese and chopped fresh parsley over the top of the vegetables.

5. Serve the Hummus and Veggie Plate immediately, with the vegetables and hummus available for dipping.

Tips:
• Use a variety of colorful vegetables for a visually appealing presentation.
• Adjust the amounts of each vegetable to your taste preferences.
• Serve with pita bread or whole grain crackers on the side.
• For extra flavor, try drizzling a bit of olive oil or balsamic glaze over the vegetables.

101. Egg and Veggie Scramble

Ingredient:

• 6 large eggs
• 2 tbsp milk or unsweetened almond milk
• 1/4 tsp salt
• 1/4 tsp black pepper
• 1 tbsp olive oil
• 1/2 cup diced bell pepper
• 1/2 cup diced onion
• 1 cup chopped spinach or kale
• 2 tbsp shredded cheddar cheese (optional)

Instructions:

1. In a medium bowl, whisk together the eggs, milk, salt, and pepper until well combined.

2. Heat the olive oil in a large non•stick skillet over medium heat.

3. Add the diced bell pepper and onion to the skillet. Cook for 3•4 minutes, stirring occasionally, until the vegetables are softened.

4. Add the chopped spinach or kale to the skillet and cook for 1•2 minutes until wilted.

5. Pour the egg mixture into the skillet and use a spatula to gently push and fold the eggs as they cook, creating soft, fluffy curds.

6. Continue cooking the scramble, folding occasionally, for 2•3 minutes until the eggs are cooked through but still moist.

7. Remove from heat and stir in the shredded cheddar cheese, if using.

8. Serve the egg and veggie scramble immediately, while hot.

102. Chicken and Vegetable Stew

Ingredient:

• 1 lb boneless, skinless chicken breasts, cut into 1•inch cubes
• 2 tbsp olive oil
• 1 onion, diced
• 3 cloves garlic, minced
• 2 carrots, peeled and sliced
• 2 celery stalks, sliced
• 1 cup diced potatoes
• 1 cup frozen peas
• 4 cups low•sodium chicken broth
• 1 tsp dried thyme
• 1 tsp dried rosemary
• 1/2 tsp salt
• 1/4 tsp black pepper

Instructions:

1. In a large pot or Dutch oven, heat the olive oil over medium•high heat.

2. Add the cubed chicken to the pot and cook for 3•4 minutes, stirring occasionally, until lightly browned.

3. Add the diced onion and minced garlic to the pot. Cook for 2•3 minutes, stirring frequently, until the onion is translucent.

4. Stir in the sliced carrots, celery, diced potatoes, and frozen peas. Pour in the chicken broth and add the dried thyme, rosemary, salt, and black pepper.

5. Bring the stew to a boil, then reduce the heat to medium•low and let it simmer for 20•25 minutes, or until the vegetables are tender and the chicken is cooked through.

6. Taste and adjust seasoning as needed.

7. Serve the Chicken and Vegetable Stew hot, garnished with additional fresh herbs if desired.

Tips:
• You can use boneless, skinless chicken thighs instead of breasts for more flavor.
• Add other vegetables like green beans, corn, or mushrooms to the stew.
• Serve the stew with crusty bread or over mashed potatoes for a heartier meal.

103. Baked Salmon with Brown Rice

Ingredient:

• 4 (6 oz) salmon fillets
• 2 tbsp olive oil
• 1 tsp garlic powder
• 1 tsp dried dill
• 1/2 tsp salt
• 1/4 tsp black pepper
• 2 cups cooked brown rice
• 1 cup steamed broccoli florets
• 2 tbsp lemon juice

Instructions:

1. Preheat oven to 400°F. Line a baking sheet with parchment paper.

2. Place the salmon fillets on the prepared baking sheet. Drizzle with the olive oil and sprinkle with the garlic powder, dried dill, salt, and black pepper.

3. Bake the salmon for 12•15 minutes, or until it flakes easily with a fork and reaches an internal temperature of 145°F.

4. While the salmon is baking, prepare the brown rice and steam the broccoli florets.

5. Once the salmon is cooked, divide the brown rice and steamed broccoli evenly among 4 plates. Top each plate with a baked salmon fillet.

6. Drizzle the lemon juice over the salmon and serve immediately.

Tip:
• For extra flavor, you can also top the salmon with lemon slices or chopped fresh parsley before baking.

104. Greek Yogurt with Fresh Fruit

Ingredient:

- 1 cup plain Greek yogurt
- 1 cup mixed fresh fruit (such as berries, sliced peaches, mango, etc.)
- 1•2 tbsp honey (optional)
- 1 tbsp chopped nuts or granola (optional)

Instructions:

1. Spoon the Greek yogurt into a serving bowl or individual bowls.

2. Top the yogurt with the mixed fresh fruit.

3. If desired, drizzle the honey over the fruit and yogurt.

4. Sprinkle the chopped nuts or granola over the top, if using.

That's it! This simple and healthy snack or breakfast is ready to enjoy.

Tips:
- Use a variety of fresh, seasonal fruits for the best flavor and nutrition.
- Choose plain, unsweetened Greek yogurt for more protein and less added sugar.
- Add a sprinkle of cinnamon or a squeeze of lemon juice for extra flavor.
- For a creamier texture, blend the yogurt and fruit together.
- Make it ahead of time and refrigerate for a quick and easy breakfast or snack.

105. Turkey and Veggie Wrap

Ingredient:

- 2 whole wheat tortillas or wraps
- 4 oz sliced turkey breast
- 1/2 cup shredded lettuce
- 1/2 cup diced tomatoes
- 1/4 cup sliced cucumber
- 2 tbsp hummus
- 1 tbsp crumbled feta cheese (optional)
- 1 tsp olive oil
- 1 tsp balsamic vinegar
- Salt and pepper to taste

Instructions:

1. Lay the tortillas or wraps out flat on a clean surface.

2. Divide the sliced turkey evenly between the two wraps, placing it in the center.

3. Top the turkey with the shredded lettuce, diced tomatoes, and sliced cucumber.

4. Spread 1 tbsp of hummus over the vegetables on each wrap.

5. Sprinkle the crumbled feta cheese over the top, if using.

6. Drizzle the olive oil and balsamic vinegar over the fillings.

7. Season with salt and pepper to taste.

8. Fold the bottom of the wrap up over the filling, then fold in the sides and continue rolling up tightly into a wrap.

9. Serve immediately or wrap in parchment paper or foil to enjoy later.

Tips:
- Use your favorite vegetables like bell peppers, shredded carrots, or sprouts.
- Try different types of cheese like cheddar or provolone.
- Add a spread like mustard or avocado for extra flavor.
- For a heartier wrap, add a small amount of cooked quinoa or brown rice.

106. Cottage Cheese with Cherry Tomatoes

Ingredient:

• 1 cup low•fat or non•fat cottage cheese
• 1 cup cherry tomatoes, halved
• 1 tbsp chopped fresh basil (or 1 tsp dried basil)
• 1 tsp olive oil
• 1/4 tsp salt
• 1/8 tsp black pepper

Instructions:

1. In a small bowl, combine the cottage cheese, halved cherry tomatoes, chopped fresh basil, olive oil, salt, and black pepper. Stir gently to mix.

2. Serve immediately or refrigerate until ready to serve.

That's it! This simple and healthy snack or light meal is ready to enjoy.

Tips:
• Use different types of tomatoes, such as grape or heirloom, for variety.
• Add a sprinkle of grated Parmesan cheese or crumbled feta for extra flavor.
• For a heartier meal, serve the cottage cheese and tomatoes over a bed of mixed greens or with whole grain crackers.
• Experiment with different fresh herbs like parsley, chives, or oregano.
• Drizzle a bit of balsamic glaze or lemon juice over the top for a flavor boost.

Cottage cheese is a great source of protein, and the cherry tomatoes provide vitamins, minerals, and antioxidants. This dish makes for a quick, nutritious, and satisfying snack or light meal.

107. Baked Sweet Potato Chips

Ingredient:

• 2 medium sweet potatoes, washed and sliced into 1/8•inch thick rounds
• 1 tbsp olive oil
• 1/2 tsp salt
• 1/4 tsp black pepper

Instructions:

1. Preheat your oven to 375°F. Line two large baking sheets with parchment paper.

2. In a large bowl, toss the sweet potato slices with the olive oil, salt, and black pepper until evenly coated.

3. Arrange the sweet potato slices in a single layer on the prepared baking sheets, making sure they are not overlapping.

4. Bake for 15•20 minutes, flipping the slices halfway through, until the chips are crispy and lightly browned.

5. Remove the baking sheets from the oven and let the chips cool completely on the sheets. They will continue to crisp up as they cool.

6. Once cooled, transfer the baked sweet potato chips to an airtight container or resealable bag for storage.

Tips:
• Use a mandoline slicer or sharp knife to get the sweet potato slices as thin and even as possible for best results.
• Adjust the baking time as needed, keeping a close eye on the chips to prevent burning.
• Experiment with different seasonings like garlic powder, paprika, or cayenne pepper.
• Store the baked chips in a single layer to maintain their crispness.

108. Beef and Veggie Kabobs

Ingredient:

• 1 lb beef sirloin or tenderloin, cut into 1•inch cubes
• 1 red bell pepper, cut into 1•inch pieces
• 1 yellow bell pepper, cut into 1•inch pieces
• 1 red onion, cut into 1•inch pieces
• 8 oz mushrooms, halved
• 2 tbsp olive oil
• 2 tbsp balsamic vinegar
• 1 tsp dried oregano
• 1/2 tsp salt
• 1/4 tsp black pepper

Instructions:

1. Preheat your grill or grill pan to medium•high heat.

2. In a large bowl, combine the beef cubes, bell pepper pieces, onion pieces, and mushrooms.

3. In a small bowl, whisk together the olive oil, balsamic vinegar, oregano, salt, and black pepper.

4. Pour the marinade over the beef and vegetables and toss to coat everything evenly.

5. Thread the marinated beef and vegetables onto skewers, alternating the ingredients.

6. Grill the kabobs for 12•15 minutes, turning occasionally, until the beef is cooked through and the vegetables are tender.

7. Serve the Beef and Veggie Kabobs immediately, while hot.

Tips:
• Soak wooden skewers in water for 30 minutes before using to prevent them from burning.
• Use a variety of colorful vegetables like zucchini, cherry tomatoes, or pineapple chunks.
• Marinate the kabobs for 30 minutes to 1 hour for more flavor.
• Serve the kabobs over a bed of rice or quinoa for a complete meal.

109. Lentil and Quinoa Salad

Ingredient:

- 1 cup uncooked quinoa, rinsed
- 1 cup cooked lentils
- 1 cup diced cucumber
- 1 cup cherry tomatoes, halved
- 1/2 cup diced red onion
- 1/4 cup chopped fresh parsley
- 2 tbsp olive oil
- 2 tbsp lemon juice
- 1 tsp Dijon mustard
- 1/2 tsp salt
- 1/4 tsp black pepper

Instructions:

1. Cook the quinoa according to package instructions. Fluff with a fork and let cool.

2. In a large bowl, combine the cooked quinoa, cooked lentils, diced cucumber, cherry tomatoes, red onion, and chopped parsley.

3. In a small bowl, whisk together the olive oil, lemon juice, Dijon mustard, salt, and black pepper to make the dressing.

4. Pour the dressing over the quinoa and lentil mixture and toss gently to coat.

5. Refrigerate the salad for at least 30 minutes to allow the flavors to meld.

6. Serve chilled or at room temperature.

Tips:
- Use canned or pre•cooked lentils to save time.
- Add other vegetables like bell peppers, carrots, or zucchini if desired.
- For extra protein, top with grilled chicken or crumbled feta cheese.
- This salad can be made a day in advance and stored in the refrigerator.

110. Chicken and Avocado Bowl

Ingredient:

• 1 lb boneless, skinless chicken breasts, grilled or baked and diced
• 1 ripe avocado, diced
• 1 cup cooked quinoa
• 1 cup cherry tomatoes, halved
• 1/2 cup diced cucumber
• 1/4 cup diced red onion
• 2 tbsp chopped fresh cilantro
• 2 tbsp lime juice
• 1 tbsp olive oil
• 1/2 tsp salt
• 1/4 tsp black pepper

Instructions:

1. In a large bowl, combine the diced grilled or baked chicken, diced avocado, cooked quinoa, cherry tomatoes, diced cucumber, and diced red onion.

2. In a small bowl, whisk together the chopped cilantro, lime juice, olive oil, salt, and black pepper to make the dressing.

3. Pour the dressing over the chicken and avocado mixture and gently toss to coat everything evenly.

4. Serve the Chicken and Avocado Bowl immediately, or refrigerate until ready to serve.

Tips:
• Use leftover or rotisserie chicken to save time.
• Substitute brown rice or cauliflower rice for the quinoa if desired.
• Add other veggies like bell peppers, corn, or black beans.
• Top with crumbled feta or shredded cheddar cheese.
• For a spicy kick, add a pinch of cayenne pepper or chopped jalapeño.

This Chicken and Avocado Bowl is a nutritious and flavorful meal that's perfect for lunch or dinner. Enjoy!

111. Apple and Cheddar Wrap

Ingredient:

• 2 whole wheat tortillas or wraps
• 2 oz sliced cheddar cheese
• 1 medium apple, thinly sliced
• 2 tbsp honey mustard or Dijon mustard
• 1 tbsp chopped walnuts (optional)

Instructions:

1. Lay the tortillas or wraps out flat on a clean surface.

2. Divide the sliced cheddar cheese evenly between the two wraps, placing it in the center.

3. Top the cheese with the thinly sliced apple.

4. Drizzle the honey mustard or Dijon mustard over the apple slices.

5. Sprinkle the chopped walnuts over the top, if using.

6. Fold the bottom of the wrap up over the filling, then fold in the sides and continue rolling up tightly into a wrap.

7. Serve immediately or wrap in parchment paper or foil to enjoy later.

Tips:
• Use your favorite type of apple, such as Gala, Honeycrisp, or Fuji.
• For extra crunch, add a handful of baby spinach or arugula.
• Substitute goat cheese or feta for the cheddar cheese.
• Drizzle a bit of balsamic glaze over the apple slices for added flavor.
• Swap the honey mustard for regular mustard or a fruit•based spread.

This Apple and Cheddar Wrap makes for a delicious and satisfying lunch or snack. The combination of sweet apple, savory cheese, and tangy mustard creates a delightful flavor profile.

112. Grilled Tuna Salad

Ingredient:

• 4 (6 oz) tuna steaks
• 2 tbsp olive oil
• 1 tsp lemon pepper seasoning
• 8 cups mixed greens (such as spinach, arugula, and romaine)
• 1 cup cherry tomatoes, halved
• 1/2 cup diced cucumber
• 1/4 cup sliced red onion
• 2 tbsp crumbled feta cheese
• 2 tbsp balsamic vinaigrette

Instructions:

1. Preheat your grill or grill pan to medium·high heat.

2. Brush the tuna steaks with the olive oil and sprinkle them evenly with the lemon pepper seasoning.

3. Grill the tuna steaks for 3·4 minutes per side, or until they reach your desired level of doneness. Transfer the grilled tuna to a cutting board and let it rest for 5 minutes.

4. In a large salad bowl, combine the mixed greens, cherry tomatoes, diced cucumber, and sliced red onion.

5. Slice the grilled tuna steaks into thin strips and add them to the salad.

6. Sprinkle the crumbled feta cheese over the top of the salad.

7. Drizzle the balsamic vinaigrette over the salad and toss gently to coat.

8. Serve the Grilled Tuna Salad immediately.

Tips:
• Use fresh, high·quality tuna steaks for the best flavor and texture.
• Adjust the cooking time for the tuna based on your desired level of doneness.
• Substitute other vegetables, such as bell peppers or avocado, to customize the salad.
• For extra protein, add a hard·boiled egg or some chickpeas.
• Use a different type of cheese, such as goat cheese or shredded cheddar.

113. Vegetable and Bean Stew

Ingredient:

• 2 tbsp olive oil
• 1 onion, diced
• 3 cloves garlic, minced
• 2 carrots, peeled and sliced
• 2 celery stalks, sliced
• 1 red bell pepper, diced
• 1 zucchini, diced
• 1 (15 oz) can diced tomatoes
• 1 (15 oz) can kidney beans, drained and rinsed
• 1 (15 oz) can chickpeas, drained and rinsed
• 4 cups low•sodium vegetable broth
• 1 tsp dried thyme
• 1 tsp dried oregano
• 1/2 tsp salt
• 1/4 tsp black pepper
• 2 tbsp chopped fresh parsley (for garnish)

Instructions:

1. In a large pot or Dutch oven, heat the olive oil over medium heat.

2. Add the diced onion and minced garlic to the pot. Cook for 2•3 minutes, stirring frequently, until the onion is translucent.

3. Stir in the sliced carrots, celery, diced bell pepper, and diced zucchini. Cook for 5•7 minutes, stirring occasionally, until the vegetables start to soften.

4. Pour in the diced tomatoes, kidney beans, and chickpeas. Add the vegetable broth, dried thyme, dried oregano, salt, and black pepper.

5. Bring the stew to a boil, then reduce the heat to medium•low and let it simmer for 20•25 minutes, or until the vegetables are tender.

6. Taste and adjust seasoning as needed.

7. Serve the Vegetable and Bean Stew hot, garnished with the chopped fresh parsley.

114. Turkey and Spinach Wrap

Ingredient:

• 2 whole wheat tortillas or wraps
• 4 oz sliced turkey breast
• 1 cup fresh spinach leaves
• 1/2 avocado, sliced
• 2 tbsp hummus
• 1 tbsp shredded cheddar cheese
• 1 tsp olive oil
• 1 tsp balsamic vinegar
• Salt and pepper to taste

Instructions:

1. Lay the tortillas or wraps out flat on a clean surface.

2. Divide the sliced turkey evenly between the two wraps, placing it in the center.

3. Top the turkey with the fresh spinach leaves, sliced avocado, and hummus.

4. Sprinkle the shredded cheddar cheese over the top.

5. Drizzle the olive oil and balsamic vinegar over the fillings.

6. Season with salt and pepper to taste.

7. Fold the bottom of the wrap up over the filling, then fold in the sides and continue rolling up tightly into a wrap.

8. Serve immediately or wrap in parchment paper or foil to enjoy later.

Tips:
• Use your favorite type of turkey, such as smoked or roasted.
• Substitute other greens like arugula or kale for the spinach.
• Add other veggies like sliced cucumber, bell peppers, or shredded carrots.
• Try different types of cheese like feta or Swiss.
• For extra flavor, spread a thin layer of mustard or pesto on the tortilla before assembling.

115. Baked Chicken Alfredo with Whole Wheat Pasta

Ingredient:

- 8 oz whole wheat pasta (such as penne or fettuccine)
- 1 lb boneless, skinless chicken breasts, cubed
- 2 tbsp olive oil
- 1 garlic clove, minced
- 2 cups low•fat milk
- 2 tbsp all•purpose flour
- 1 cup grated Parmesan cheese
- 1/2 tsp salt
- 1/4 tsp black pepper
- 1/4 cup panko breadcrumbs
- 2 tbsp chopped fresh parsley (optional)

Instructions:

1. Preheat your oven to 375°F. Grease a 9x13 inch baking dish.

2. Cook the whole wheat pasta according to package instructions. Drain and set aside.

3. In a large skillet, heat the olive oil over medium•high heat. Add the cubed chicken and minced garlic. Cook for 5•7 minutes, stirring occasionally, until the chicken is lightly browned.

4. In a saucepan, whisk together the milk and flour. Bring the mixture to a simmer and cook for 2•3 minutes, stirring constantly, until thickened.

5. Remove the sauce from heat and stir in 1/2 cup of the Parmesan cheese, salt, and black pepper.

6. In the prepared baking dish, layer the cooked pasta, chicken, and Parmesan sauce. Top with the remaining 1/2 cup Parmesan cheese and the panko breadcrumbs.

7. Bake for 20•25 minutes, or until the top is golden brown and the sauce is bubbly.

8. Remove from the oven and let stand for 5 minutes. Garnish with the chopped fresh parsley, if desired.

Congratulations on completing ***"Healthy Cookbook for Teen Boys: Boost Your Energy with 115+ Balanced and Flavorful Dishes"!*** You've taken an important step toward fueling your body with nutritious and delicious meals that support your active lifestyle as a teenage boy.

What You've Accomplished

Throughout this cookbook, you've explored over 115 recipes designed to provide you with the essential nutrients your body needs to thrive. From energizing breakfasts and satisfying lunches to wholesome dinners and nutritious snacks, each recipe has been crafted to help you maintain peak performance, whether you're hitting the field, studying hard, or simply enjoying time with friends.

Beyond the Kitchen

Cooking isn't just about preparing food—it's about learning valuable life skills that will serve you well into the future. By mastering the art of cooking nutritious meals, you've gained independence, confidence, and the ability to make informed choices about your health and well-being.

Keep Exploring

Your journey with food and cooking doesn't end here. Continue to experiment with the recipes in this book, try out new ingredients, and customize dishes to suit your tastes and preferences. Cooking is a creative process, and each meal you prepare is an opportunity to expand your culinary skills and discover new flavors.

Share Your Passion

As you continue on your culinary adventure, don't forget to share your love for cooking with others. Invite friends and family to enjoy the meals you've prepared, and inspire them to embrace healthier eating habits too. Food has a unique way of bringing people together, creating memories, and fostering relationships.

Final Thoughts

Thank you for choosing "Healthy Cookbook for Teen Boys: Boost Your Energy with 115+ Balanced and Flavorful Dishes" as your guide to nutritious and delicious eating. We hope this cookbook has empowered you to take charge of your health and wellness through the joy of cooking. Here's to many more flavorful meals and a lifetime of good health. Happy cooking!